I0455001

Hormones
Working for You

By Walter Parks
CreateSpace Edition
Copyright 2012
UnKnownTruths
Publishing Company

UnKnownTruths
Publishing Company
8815 Conroy Windermere Rd. Ste 190
Orlando, FL 32835

My Blog

My Website

Other titles by Walter Parks for Kindle:

Jesus the Missing Years

Atlantis the Eyewitnesses

Immortal Again

Aging is a Treatable Disease

Paranormal Portal to a Parallel Universe

Alligator Attack!

The Devil Takes the Bodies

Caribbean Ghost, Genetic Memory Comes Alive

Clan of the Bigfoot

The Body Returns, Corpus de Licti

I Look Marvelous, Skin Care Guide

Indian Massacre in Orlando

Who the Hell is Satan

Treasure Hunt, Finding Solomon's Temple Treasure

Ancient Secrets

The Birth of Jesus, A New Christian Holiday

Finding the Soul, Surviving Death

Contents

Introduction

Medical science and the unraveling of the human genome have, and are, providing us with great insights into how our bodies work and how we are susceptible to diseases and the aging process.

Our new understandings now allow us to significantly increase our healthy longevity. And when we take advantages of these new findings we make ourselves available to take advantages of the even newer technologies being developed.

There are a dozen or so mechanisms of aging that have been theorized over time. The author believes that there are seven basic causes that combine to make us age:

1. Free radicals and other ashes of our metabolism, and environmental toxins build up in our cells and cause the cells to die without being able to reproduce themselves as they would normally do when you are younger.

2. Our endocrine system ceases to secrete sufficient quantities of certain enzymes and hormones to keep up with the cell's battles with the build up of contaminants.

3. Our cells lose their ability to divide, and replace themselves because they use up their allotted number of divisions (reach their Hayflick Limits).

4. Stress causes secretion of excessive cortisol which does significant damage.

5. Some of us have inherited flawed genes that cause, or allow malfunctions.

6. Deficiencies in our diet limit the materials necessary for the cells to cleanse and repair themselves. Excesses in our diets adversely affect certain chemical reactions.

7. Lack of exercise causes atrophy of critical muscles that result in chemical imbalances and loss of strength and agility which makes us prone to accidents.

All animals studied to date share these same causes of aging that they and we have inherited from our common evolution.

The purpose of this book is to describe item 2 above which is basically our hormones. See other books that describe the other causes of aging at UnknownTruths.com.

Our hormones regulate and control most of the functions of our bodies. Testosterone and estrogen, the major sex hormones in men and women respectively, give us the urge and ability to reproduce and continue the survival of our species.

But once we're past our reproductive prime, our hormone levels drop. This results in a lack of sex drive, insomnia, impotence, weight gain, and countless other potential health problems that significantly decreases our quality of your life.

So we see that our hormone system was designed primarily for reproduction for the survival of the species. Our bodies produce high quantities of certain hormones and enzymes during our youth. These give us our youthful vitality, strength, and endurance. They help in the battles against free radicals and they help provide nutrients for cell repair. They keep our cells cleansed of the ashes of metabolism and environmental toxins.

As long as our bodies produce sufficient quantities of these enzymes and hormones, we stay young. But we, and all plants and animals were designed to stay healthy until we have reproduced and reared our young. Mother Nature has little interest in us after we have passed our genes on to the next generation.

As we age past our prime reproductive years we are no longer capable of producing sufficient quantities of the enzymes and hormones required to keep our cells "young and fit." With too little of these substances, our cells begin to lose their battles against the free radicals and other destructive elements.

The cells begin to age, and die. The organs of which they are a part become ineffective. We become frail, we die.

But we can now do something about our hormones.

To make sure you are around when new health discoveries are proven and available, you need to under your hormones and what they do for you and what you can do to keep them functioning.

Chapter 1
Human Growth Hormone (HGH)

Human Growth Hormone (HGH) is the master hormone of the body and is therefore the principle hormone in anti-aging and other hormone replacement therapies (HRT) and hormone precursor therapies (HPT).

HGH is a protein hormone, not a steroid. The somatotropic cells of the anterior lobe of the pituitary gland secrete it. Its technical name is somatotropin. It is secreted in pulses throughout the 24-hour day, with the major secretions occurring during the beginning phases of sleep.

HGH directs and supports the other hormones and thereby affects all glands and organs in the body. HGH is the body's most essential maintenance and repair hormone. And like testosterone, described below, it has major anabolic, i.e. muscle building effects.

Adequate HGH levels are required for:

Cell replacement
Tissue Repair
Healing
Bone Strength
Brain function
Organ integrity
Enzyme protection
Integrity of hair nails and skin
Re-activation of telomerase genes.

Our chief problem with HGH and several of the key hormones is that the body's natural secretion of hormones rapidly declines with age. By 60, we have less than 40% of the values we had at 20. The following chart shows the decreases for 3 of the key hormones. So we lose the benefits of key hormones as we age.

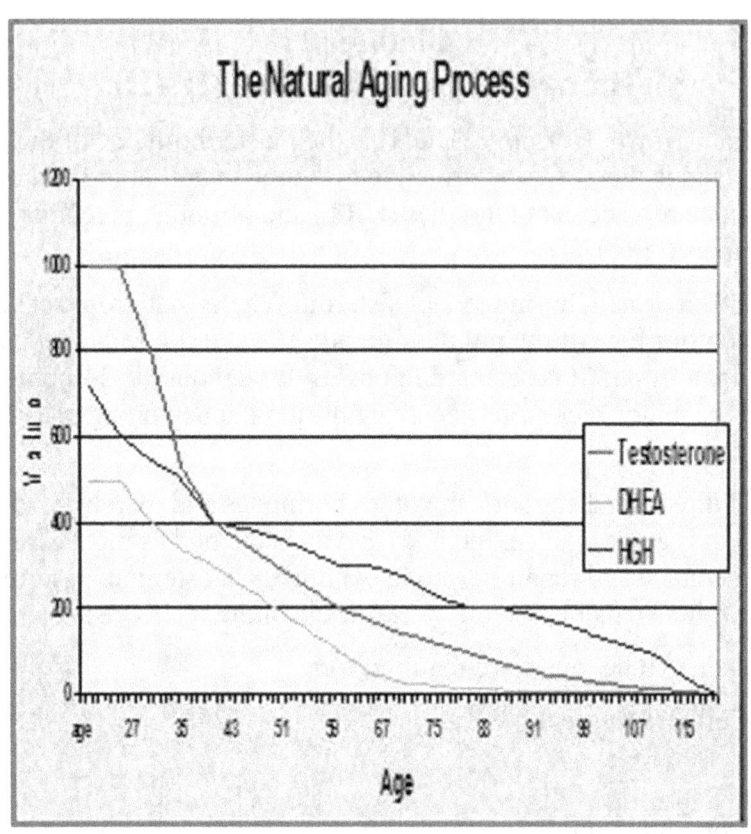

It should be noted that **HGH** is difficult to measure because of its variability during each 24-hour period. It is therefore measured indirectly by measuring insulin-like growth factor-l (IGF-l). IGF-1 is typically between 300 and 450 ng/nl (nanograms per milliliter of blood) for healthy young adults.

It declines with **HGH** as we age, at the rate of about 10 to 15 percent per decade. In older people it therefore ranges from 30 to 200. Values below 350 are considered a deficiency by many in the anti-aging community.

1) HGH History and Tests

HGH was discovered in the 1920's and first used in 1958 on a growth- stunted boy. He grew taller and since then **HGH** has become the common treatment for this disorder.

Initially, **HGH** was only available from cadavers. In 1985 Genentech spliced human DNA into bacteria and the genetically engineered bacteria began producing **HGH** at an affordable price. Eli Lilly engineered a more exact replica of **HGH** with their genetic splicing of human genes in bacteria. This produced an HGH of the precise 191 amino acids produced by normal humans – versus the 190 amino acids of the earlier synthetic. Eli Lilly is now the leader in **HGH** supply.

The limitations imposed by cadaver sources were quickly eliminated and tests of **HGH** effectiveness were conducted by Dr. Rudman in 1989.

During a six month test of 12 men aged 61-81 (against a control group of 9 men), the men lost 14.4% of their body fat and gained 8.8% lean body mass. Their skin thickened, their bone density increased and their livers and spleens increased to youthful sizes.

Dr. Rudman showed that **HGH** could change flabby, frail old men aged 61- 81 back to their previous biological ages of 41-61. In effect, he reversed their ages by 20 years, over a 6-month period. He concluded:

"The overall deterioration of the body

that comes with growing old is not inevitable."

In his follow-on six month study with the same men, their muscle mass increased an additional 6% (over the original 8.8%), and they lost an additional 15% fat (after the original 14.4% loss).

Others have repeated Dr. Rudman's tests and got similar results. There was a cry for the FDA to approve it as an anti-aging therapy. But, the FDA only approved it for the stunted-growth children.

Nevertheless, it hit the black-market and began to be widely used by bodybuilders.

Then in 1991, Texas businessman Howard Turney opened El Dorado Rejuvenation Clinic in Mexico - beyond control of the FDA.

Then in 1994, Dr. Edmund Chein found a loophole (he was also a lawyer) in the FDA restriction. He went to court and argued that since the FDA had approved **HGH** for stunted-growth disorder - then a certified physician should be able to prescribe it for any purpose he sees fit. He won his argument and opened his Palm Springs Life Extension Institute in California.

He has since treated thousands of people between the ages of 31 and 92 to slow, stop, or reverse their aging. He has reversed the aging of most. And, he reports that he has had **no significant adverse side effects during any of his operations.**

Chein's results in increased muscle mass were 10.0% and 8.0% increase for two six month periods, which are similar to Dr. Rudman's results.

UK researchers duplicated Rudman's and Chein's results. And, Dr. Bengtsson of Sweden showed vastly improved energy levels and improved mood.

The French - Dr. Thierry Hertogh - showed that his patients experienced a 23% to 30% reduction in the size of their "love handles."

HGH makes fat more available as a fuel. Fat cells have hormone receptors that trigger a host of enzymatic reactions when **HGH** is present.

HGH has also been shown to enhance the effectiveness of the immune system. One major way it does this is to increase the thymus gland's output of T-cells (that destroy invading "germs"). This is especially important for people over 40. The thymus normally shrinks to a "raisin" by age 40. (See: Thymus Factors in a later section).

Tests also indicate that **HGH** can reverse heart disease by thickening the walls of the weakened ventricles.

Tests have shown that **HGH** improves LDL/HDL cholesterol ratios. It can prevent osteoporosis - or if taken after osteoporosis onset - it can reverse it. It can improve vision, increase clarity of thought, improve - or restore - sexual functions, and re-grow hair.

Dr. Sam Boxas of Switzerland uses **HGH** to treat muscular sclerosis, lupus, Alzheimer's, Lou Gehrig's disease, and even AIDS. And, as unbelievable as it sounds, he says: "We are healing just about everything."

He is effectively reversing aging.

Several doctors have reported that HGH has resulted in their patients showing a marked progressiveness towards homeostasis; i.e. body balance. Everyone experienced higher metabolism and more youthful body chemistry. Their DHEA was generally up by 33 % and the male's testosterone levels up an average of 18.5%. Cholesterol was down an average of 14.8% and triglycerides were down 31%.

The patients generally reported the following qualitative improvements:

Weight down
Muscle increase
Energy up
Libido up
Skin rejuvenation
Hair color return
Greater hair density
Improved mental stability
There were no significant adverse side effects reported. These early tests with HGH strongly indicated that **HGH could restore youth -safely.**

2) Benefits of HGH HRT and HPT

The early tests plus the many follow-on tests have shown that **HGH** HRT and HPT can provide the following benefits:

Improved immune function
Accelerates wound healing
Strengthen bones
Reverse osteoporosis
Reverse muscle wasting
Increase muscle mass
Decrease fat
Eliminate cellulite
Reduce appetite
Increase exercise performance
Lower blood pressure
Lower bad cholesterol
Increase good HDL
Lower triglycerides
Increase cardiac output
Restore the size of heart, liver, pancreas, kidneys, spleen, and other organs that had shrunk with age
Enhance collagen synthesis and repair
Provide tighter, more hydrated, smoother, thicker skin
Improve brain function
Improve cognitive abilities
Improve memory and concentration
Grow neuron dendrites to repair brain injury or treat disease
Improve vision
Provide higher energy levels
Achieve less fatigue and less depression
Reduce stress levels
Elevate mood
Improve quality of deep sleep
Enhance sexuality, drive and performance
Reduce accumulation of lipofuscins
Prevent chronic, degenerative diseases

Reverse the effects of aging.

Dr. Ronald Klatz, President of the American Academy of Anti-Aging, and author of the book: **"Grow Young with HGH"** summarizes the benefits of **HGH** replacement therapy:

"HGH is the ultimate anti-aging therapy. It affects every cell in the body, rejuvenating the skin and bones, regenerating the heart, liver, lung, and kidneys, bringing organ and tissue function back to youthful levels. It is the most effective anti-obesity agent ever discovered, revving up the metabolism to youthful levels, re-sculpturing the body by selectively reducing the fat in the waist, abdomen, hips, thighs, and at the same time increasing muscle mass. It may be the most powerful aphrodisiac ever discovered, reviving flagging sexuality and potency in men and women. It is cosmetic surgery in a bottle, smoothing out facial wrinkles; restoring the elasticity, thickness and contours of youthful skin; reversing the loss of extra cellular water that makes old people look like dried-up old prunes. It has healing powers that close ulcerated wounds and re-grow burned skin. It reverses the insomnia of later life, restoring "slow wave" or the deepest level of sleep. And, it is a mood elevator, lifting the spirit along with the body, bringing back a zest for life that many people thought was long gone."

Dr. Edmund Chein, one of the first providers of **HGH** replacement therapy is more succinct:

"It's a slam dunk!

This (HGH) is 100% effective!"

3) HGH and the Immune System

If there is one aspect of our metabolism that simply must function effectively to ensure one's survival, it is the immune system. It has to defend us against the nasty world of microbes and viruses as well as parasites that are continuously invading our bodies. We survive their assault when our immune system works optimally.

But, as we age, so does our immune system. One of the major glands of our immune system is our thymus. In childhood, this gland creates T-lymphocytes - the specialized cells that eliminate bacteria, viruses and foreign matter from our bodies.

In late childhood, the thymus is the size of a plum, but at puberty it begins to shrink. By the time we reach old age it's no larger than a small raisin.

This atrophication of the thymus parallels the decline of our immune system.

HGH can regenerate the thymus and restore our immune system to near the optimum function that it had when we were twelve years old. The statisticians have shown that this is the age we are least likely to die from disease.

Tests on dogs in 1980 showed that when growth hormone replacement was instituted: "The thymuses of growth hormone treated dogs regenerated, resembling thymic tissue of young dogs."

In 1991, David Khansari and Thomas Gustad of North Dakota State University completed a long-term study on mice. They divided 52 mice that had reached the age of senescence (old age) into two equal groups. One group was given growth hormone for 13 weeks. Most of these members were still living after all the members of the control group had died. It was also noted that the growth hormone treated mice had T-cell counts comparable to those of young mice. With their newly empowered immune systems, they had lived beyond the limits of normal mouse longevity.

Scientists at the University of New Mexico School of Medicine took twelve older women in relatively good health, but with low **HGH** levels, and gave six of them **HGH** for fourteen days. The six treated women experienced a 20% increase in their T- cell activity compared to the untreated six.

**HGH can obviously regenerate the thymus gland
and vastly improve the immune system.**

4) HGH and the Brain

HGH is one of the very few substances that cross the blood-brain barrier.

Tests have shown that there are receptor sights for **HGH** in numerous parts of the brain - including the hypothalamus, the pituitary, and the hippocampus. The receptors in the hippocampus are of particular interest because this is a part of the brain that significantly controls cognitive functions and memory.

This recognition has made **HGH** a source of hope in treating Alzheimer's disease and other mental and memory dementia of our aging population.

One third to one half of all 85 year olds are at least in the early stages of Alzheimer's disease. Dr. Chaovanee Aroonsakul, M.D. of the Alzheimer's and Parkinson's disease Diagnostic and Treatment Center in Naperville, Illinois, has reported noticeable improvements after treatment with **HGH** in both these conditions as well as in patients suffering other forms of senile dementia.

In a study of over three hundred patients, Dr. Aroonsakul reported consistently lower levels of **HGH** in patients with Parkinson's and multiple sclerosis, as well as stroke patients, and found "profound deficiency" of HGH in Alzheimer's patients.

Dr. Aroonsakul has reported some improvement in Alzheimer's patients after several years of continuous **HGH** therapy. She believes that **HGH** improves cerebral blood flow, revitalizes neuronal dendrites and axons, and enhances repair of protein in the brain, causing an increase in the formation of RNA and DNA.

5) HGH and the Bones

Tens of millions of Americans suffer serious, crippling damage to their bones that lead more elderly people to nursing homes than any other cause.

We lose bone mass and density as we age because of hormonal declines. It begins in our thirties when androgen levels start to decline. **Bone is a hormonally sensitive tissue.**

The major "disease" of the bones is osteoporosis - which literally means "porous bones." It is perhaps the most expensive and debilitating disease in America.

Osteoporosis is a chronic degenerative bone disease that, over time, causes an excessive loss of bone. Osteoporosis is like a termite infestation. You don't know you have it until something breaks.

By their forties, most people lose bone at the rate of 0.5% per year. For women, this increases by a factor of ten after menopause. Many women lose a third of their bone mass before the age of 60. Half of all women have an osteoporosis fracture by the age of 70.

Twenty percent of osteoporosis patients are men - but their problems usually come later than for women.

Twenty four million Americans have osteoporosis and spend $10 billion per year treating it - or dealing with its consequences.

In the healthy young body, bones are continuously being torn down and rebuilt. Each year about 25% of a typical bone is dismantled, i.e. reabsorbed, and then replaced.

Osteoclasts are the cells that serve as the demolition crew. Osteoblasts are the reconstruction crew. Osteoblasts build new bone continuously by depositing calcium phosphate on the protein framework of existing bone.

The bones are built up to the level of their maximum density and health by the time we are in our twenties. They then begin a slight decline in our mid-thirties.

For those of us who want to live a long, healthy life - **we need a bone survival plan**.

Both **HGH** and testosterone (as described later) stimulate Osteoblasts to halt - and reverse - bone loss. **HGH** and the principal androgens - including testosterone - scavenge available calcium from the blood and put it back in the bone.

Therefore, our bone survival plan requires proper levels of dietary (or supplemental) calcium and proper levels of hormones that know how to put that calcium where it will do the most good.

This plan will vary from individual to individual depending on their individual health profile and dietary habits. As an example, those ingesting high quantities of sugar will need more calcium and hormones because sugar depletes our bodies of calcium. Salt and caffeine, each - also increase our excretion of calcium - within a few hours of consumption.

Phosphorus also adversely affects our bone health. Cola beverages that are high in caffeine, sugar, and phosphorus are absolutely the worst drinks possible for bone health.

Cola drinkers will need special doses of HGH.

6) <u>Benefits of HGH HRT and HPT</u>

Perhaps the best quantifiable summary of the benefits of **HGH HRT** is that by Dr. Chein and Dr. Terry from their six-month test of 202 people. These patients each gave personal assessments of the results of their treatments. Their personal assessments were combined with other results from tests by others - as previously described – which indicate many more benefits - and for the most part - even more important benefits. Unfortunately, however, some of the tests were not of a quantifiable nature.

Our resulting summary of the benefits of **HGH HRT** is presented in the charts.

HGH Benefits

Fitness Benefits	Percent Benefiting
Muscle Strength	88
Muscle Size	81
Higher Energy	87
Exercise Tolerance	81
Exercise Endurance	83
Triceps Strength	61
Shoulder Strength	44
Buttocks	42
Back Flexibility	53
Muscle/Fat Ratio	25
Appearance Benefits	Percent Benefiting
Fat Loss	72
Skin elasticity	73
Skin Texture	71
Skin Thickness	68
Sagging Cheeks	75
Wrinkled Face	71
Pouches Under Eyes	66
Skin Under Chin	63
Waist	40
Wrinkled Hands	42
New Hair Growth	38
Thicker Lips	25
Darkening of Gray Hair	10

Other Benefits/Percent Benefiting

Emotional Stability	83
Attitude	80
Emotional Stability	83
Immunity to Disease	73
Healing Capacity	71
Sexual Potency	76
Duration of Penile Erection	62
Memory	64
Nighttime Urination	57
Hot Flashes	58

The test subjects also reported benefits that could not adequately be statistically quantified because there was not adequate sampling:

Lower LDL
Lower Triglycerides
Lower Blood Pressure
Improved Osteoporosis Symptoms
Arthritis Relief

7) Adverse Side Effects of HGH HRT

Fluid retention was the most common side effect reported. All reported - however - that it was a very transient effect that ceased after a day or two. Even this transient effect was shown to be avoidable by starting patients at lower dosages and then ramping up to the desired dose over time.

Some patients reported acne. Ramping also eliminated this side effect.

Arthralgia (joint pain) was reported in a few cases (0.7%). Again, down ramping eliminated the problem.

Carpal tunnel syndrome was also reported in a few cases (0.5%) and was eliminated by down ramping.

Other researchers have also reported these side effects plus gynecomastia and painful cartilage growth. But in all cases reported, the doses were very much higher than the doses used and recommended by doctors working in this area.

There has also been some concern expressed by some critics that **HGH** replacement therapy could increase the probability of some cancers - especially the spreading of cancers already existing when therapy is initiated. The primary cancers of concern are breast and prostate cancers.

But, on the contrary, **tests by Dr. Terry showed that some existing cancers went into remission when HGH therapy was used!**

Dr. Terry said: "It is mind – boggling." He does not know why the remission occurred. Dr. Chein speculates that the growth hormone stimulated the immune system, increasing the natural killer cells, which effectively destroyed the cancer cells.

Another concern is that the pituitary gland may reduce its secretion of **HGH** when **HGH** is given externally, i.e. by replacement therapy. The authors also have this concern.

We have provided a tailored formula of precursor nutracuetials to prevent such gland atrophy. This formula addresses all the concerns of all the adverse side effects by the use of precursors to stimulate the body to produce its own HGH.

Dr. George Merriam at the University of Washington in Seattle conducted a study on growth hormone for the National Institute of Aging (NIA), and concluded.

> **"There is no evidence suggesting that this**
> **(growth Hormone) replacement therapy**
> **causes any unfavorable long term side effects**
> **A complete absence of side effects."**
>
> **Dr. George Merriam**

There have been no adverse side effects reported for HPT which is the therapy used with our nutracuetials.

8) HGH Levels

Men and women have about the same HGH levels.

Age	Levels*
5	2000
10	1280
20	700
30	500
40	400
50	350
60	270
70	230
80	200
90	160
100	115
110	60
120	0

* In micrograms per mili-liter of blood

9) HGH Precursors

The table depicts the precursors for **HGH.** It is best to take each of the supplements with meals, where IX signifies breakfast, 2X breakfast and dinner, and 3X all three meals. It is noted that these supplements are mixed with other supplements in proprietary formulas that include other supplements for other hormone precursors.

Supplement	Dose	Frequency
L-Arginine	1000 mg	2X1 /day
L-Ornithine	500 mg	2X1 / day
Choline	200 mg	1X1 / day
Vitamin B5	165 mg	1X1 / day
Vitamin C	1000 mg	3X1 / day
Vitamin E	400 IU	2X1 / day
Selenium	50 mcg	2X1 / day
Cysteine	500 mg	2X1 / day

L-Arginine and Ornithine are amino acids that stimulate the pituitary gland to increase its secretion of **HGH.** Both of these must be taken with antioxidants, hence the need for vitamins C and E, and for selenium all of which are antioxidants.

L-Arginine has the "side effect" that it produces better erections in men.

Choline is a very good **HGH** precursor that is also a key factor in fat metabolism. It helps burn fat. It also improves cardiac function, memory, and mood; and it helps to lower blood pressure. It generally **should not be taken with blood pressure medicine.**

Cysteine is an amino acid needed as a building block that makes the other amino acids more effective.

Vitamin B5 - also known as **pantethine** - is a coenzyme that is a very good **HGH** precursor that stimulates for increased adrenaline and thereby provides more energy.

It is noted that some doctors prescribe a combination of:

Niacin
Tyrosine
Glutathione
Methionine

As precursors for HGH, but we believe that the above recommended formulation is far more effective.

Others use somatomedin, which is a direct HGH releasing hormone. This may be more effective than the above formulation but it could cause gland atrophy therefore it is not recommend.

10) HGH Summary

Proper levels of HGH are necessary for optimum health. The benefits are enormous. However there can be significant adverse affects for HRT. Therefore it is safer to use HPT because, though it is less effective, there are essentially no adverse side effects. Tests have shown that the recommended HGH precursors, taken properly, will return HGH levels towards more youthful levels and will, at least partially, re-activate the telomerase genes and slow aging.

Chapter 2
Testosterone

Testosterone is the primary male sex hormone and is a secondary but very vital female sex hormone. Women produce it to the levels of about one tenth to one twelfth that of men.

Testosterone is produced by the testicles in men and by the ovaries in women. It builds up in boys and causes the changes of puberty; **it makes a male a male**.

Estrogen is the principal female hormone that makes a female a female, but it is testosterone that triggers some of the secondary sex changes in females at puberty, and stimulates her sex drive.

**Testosterone sets the sex drive
in both men and women.**

There are receptors for testosterone in every part of our bodies - from brain to toes. The sexual areas of our bodies, men and women, are **packed** with testosterone receptors.

When a girl reaches puberty, it is testosterone that stimulates the growth of pubic hair and underarm hair. At the same time, there are testosterone receptors in the nipples of her developing breasts and a heavy concentration in the area of her vagina and clitoris. There is little or no arousal unless testosterone flows to those regions.

Testosterone is also vitally involved in the making of protein, which in turn, forms muscle. And testosterone is a key player in the manufacturer of bone.

Testosterone improves oxygen uptake throughout the body, thus vitalizing all tissues. Testosterone helps:

Control Blood Sugar.
Regulate Cholesterol.
Maintain a Powerful Immune System.
Mental Concentration.
Improve Mood.

Protect Against Alzheimer's disease.
Partially re-activates the telomerase genes.

Testosterone levels in healthy young men range from 1000 to about 800 nanograms per deciliter (ng/dl) of blood. Women will normally have levels of 10 to 100 prior to menopause and some may have levels of as much as 10 to 50 after menopause. Most women, however, have much lower levels after menopause.

Biologically active testosterone drops rapidly with age as is shown in the previous chart. For many men, the drop after age 40 is even more drastic than the norm shown in the chart. This is generally the case for over 20% of men over the age of 50.

The female production of free testosterone drops in the same fashion as men until their ovaries shut down at menopause. Thereafter their body usually converts a small amount of testosterone from DHEA. This amount is usually insufficient for normal - youthful - body functions.

When testosterone gets below a certain level, there is a profound effect on physical health and "well being." Specific symptoms are:

Loss of libido in both sexes and inability to maintain an erection in men;
Fatigue, irritability, depressed mood;
Aches and pains in joints;
Dry skin;
Osteoporosis;
Muscle loss;
Hair loss.

The "natural" decrease in our production of testosterone can occur sooner with the presence of any of the following factors:

Illness;
Medication;
Obesity;
Lack of exercise;
Poor psychological state;

Smoking;
Excessive Alcohol;
Diabetes;
Nutritional deficiency;
Human Growth Hormone (HGH) deficiency.

1) The Male Andropause

The lower levels of free testosterone for men, whether occurring with the decrease over time as depicted in the chart, or whether resulting from the 20% or so abnormalities, eventually cause all males to experience a "male menopause." This is sometimes referred to as an "Andropause" or a "change of life" or "the male climacteric." It is not as sudden as the female menopause. It may typically occur over a period of fifteen years or so. And it starts at different times for different men: some as early as the 40's, some as late as the 80's.

Arguments as to the occurrence of the male Andropause still continue - even though Dr. Carl Heller and Dr. Gordon Myers published the first proof in the *Journal of the American Medical Association* over fifty years ago. They compared 38 men with "mid-life symptoms" with 25 healthy men. 23 of the 38 men had low testosterone levels. A 25 mg injection of testosterone was given to all the men five times per week for a period of two to four weeks. By the second week there were definite improvements in all the 23 men who had initially tested low in testosterone.

When testosterone was later withheld, their "mid-life symptoms" returned. It was concluded that the male Andropause did exist and that it could be treated with testosterone replacement. This replacement is typically referred to as Hormone Replacement Therapy (HRT).

2) Testosterone HRT and HPT for Men

Testosterone levels for optimal sex for men vary over very large ranges. The optimum level is directly related to the "normal" for the individual. Men with very high testosterone levels in their youth may experience sexual problems with drops to levels still as high as 500, while men with low levels of testosterone in their youth will have excellent sexual function at a level of 500.

Testosterone HRT may be administered by intra-muscular injections, via patches, or by the applications of creams, with the best method being dependent on the individual.

Testosterone HPT is not as fast acting or as effective as HRT. But it is safer and does not conflict with the government's effective band on HRT for anti-aging.

3) Testosterone HRT and HPT for Women

Testosterone is not just for men. Testosterone, the quintessential male hormone, is also a female hormone.

Healthy women naturally have small amounts of testosterone in their bodies. In fact, it is produced by the female reproductive organs, the ovaries.

As with estrogen and progesterone, a woman's testosterone levels drop as she ages. A woman could be diligently taking her estrogen and progesterone each day, and she may still not feel like herself. That is because she is ignoring another of her essential hormones: testosterone.

Testosterone is important in triggering some of the processes a girl undergoes during puberty.

If testosterone is not at its optimal level, the female body is still a bit out of balance. Since the goal is to truly replace all the hormones to a youthful level, testosterone must be included in the mix.

4) Female Libido Enhancement

One of testosterone's primary female functions is helping to control a woman's libido. Research also shows that testosterone levels, which fluctuate dramatically throughout the menstrual cycle, are highest just prior to ovulation. Combine this surge with the influx of progesterone, and it is no wonder that many women feel their greatest sexual drive and energy at this particular time.

Dr. Barbara Sherwin of McGill University in Montreal has studied testosterone replacement in post-menopausal women for the past 20 years. The most dramatic effect she has observed is how testosterone influences a woman's libido. With the decline in hormones at menopause, a woman's sex drive decreases. Some women lose interest in sex altogether.

But Dr. Sherwin's studies showed that women who took the testosterone regained their desire for sex and enjoyed it more. These women frequently reported that they experienced more orgasms.

86% of post-menopausal women report a decline in their libido and level of sexual activity. Although some part of this change is due to estrogenic deficiency resulting in vaginal atrophy, loss of energy, and increased depression, most of it is actually caused by a decline in androgens.

The principal areas of testosterone application, depending on the deficiencies being treated can include the levator ani - the muscle between the pubic bone and the tailbone. This muscle controls the firmness of the vaginal muscle and the muscles that control excretions.

Applications also include differing parts of the female genitalia and other skin-muscle areas for the more generalized testosterone therapy needs. Testosterone placement, and the proper doses, should be specified based on each individual's situation.

In many women, testosterone levels begin falling even before menopause sometimes resulting in a declining level of sexual interest as early as the late thirties. By the time they reach their forties or fifties many women report a marked sexual decline, sometimes even a feeling of complete sexual deadness.

Overall a woman's levels of testosterone decline by approximately 50% in the years after menopause. Perhaps half of this decline is due to the complete shutdown of testosterone production in the ovaries. Equally important, however, are the adrenal glands declining production of two other important steroids: androstenedione and DHEA. These two hormones have relatively weak androgenic action of their own, but a convenient process converts them to testosterone intra-cellular throughout the body. It is called peripheral conversion.

Those on **estrogen HRT** complain that the therapy does not bring back the sexual desires and feelings of their youth. This is generally due to **lack of testosterone**. Female testosterone levels are frequently lowered by any combination of the following:

Childbirth
Chemotherapy
Surgery (adrenal stress)
Endometriosis
Psychological trauma and depression
Birth control pills
Ovarectomy
Normal aging, including menopause

For a woman to have an optimal sex drive, Testosterone levels need to be in the range of 30 to 60 ng/dl.

Testosterone's other effects also have a payoff in terms of sexuality. If a woman has improved muscle tone, more energy, and greater general vitality, this can only enhance her responsiveness once she begins to feel the first stirrings of resurrected sexuality.

Testosterone is also needed by women to help strengthen the levator ani - the muscle between the pubic bone and the tailbone. [Remember: This muscle controls the firmness of the vaginal muscle and the muscles that control excretions.] Many older women lose control of urination and experience leakage as this muscle weakens.

Millions of women begin to suffer bladder leakage in their forties and fifties and don't know what to do about it. Most often they find that when they laugh, cough, or make some intense physical effort, urine escapes. As one patient put it, "Three sneezes and it is time for a change of underwear!"

The reason for the problem is loss of muscle tone in the muscles of the pelvic sling, the levator ani. In both men and women, these muscles are peculiarly dependent on testosterone. Women who have bladder leakage find that rubbing a small amount of testosterone cream into the area between the bottom of the vagina and the anus will strengthen those muscles, especially if combined with Kegel exercises, an easy to do program that involves periodically contracting the muscles in the pelvic area. Kegel exercises also have a highly favorable effect on sexual function in both women and men.

5) Menopausal Relief

Testosterone does more for a woman than boost her libido. In fact testosterone enhances the functions of estrogen. One of the primary uses of testosterone is for women who take estrogen and progesterone but still have no relief from severe menopausal symptoms.

When these women begin taking testosterone as well, the mood swings and irritability generally disappear.

6) Female Bone Health

As discovered in tests with male testosterone supplementation, testosterone is also instrumental in strengthening the bones and preventing osteoporosis. We have seen that estrogen can slow the destruction of bone, but not help rebuild it. Like progesterone, when testosterone is given with estrogen, the damaged bones begin to rebuild and strengthen. So rather than slowing the progression of osteoporosis, optimum hormone therapy can actually reverse it or even prevent it altogether.

7) Decreased Breast Cancer Risk

When women take testosterone in combination with their other hormones, their therapy is much more physiologic. This means that by adding testosterone to the mix, the body better accepts all the other hormones, with fewer side effects and with increased benefits.

One such benefit may be a decreased risk of breast cancer in women. Testosterone replacement is essential to a woman's overall physical and mental well-being.

8) Benefits of Testosterone HRT and HPT

Testosterone replacement therapies have been practiced for several years. In a test of 94 men in Sweden, 92% of the patients were able to return to "normal;" their bodies performed just like men that produced normal levels of testosterone.

In another test, twenty-nine male patients produced notable improvements in erectile functions, libido, and mood within eight weeks.

In another test of thirteen healthy, but elderly men, twelve experienced a return to youthful performance.

Many additional tests have been conducted throughout the world. Dr. Perring in London has treated over 800 patients and has shown a return to youthful libido and feelings of well being and youthful performance when testosterone HRT was taken in conjunction with DHEA.

Collectively, tests over the years have shown that testosterone replacement therapy can:

Cause the body to use protein to build:
    More and stronger muscles;
    Thicker skin and improved skin tone;
    Improved bone density;
Decrease the percentage of body fat;
Increase strength and endurance;
Improved mood;
Reverse joint pain;
Retard - and sometimes reverse osteoporosis;
Lower cholesterol;

Decrease risk of heart attack;
Normalize abnormal electrocardiograms;
Lower insulin requirements in diabetics;
Improve retinopathy;
Eliminate dry skin;
Protect against autoimmune diseases;
Stimulate growth of certain organs;
Regulate production of prostaglandin that keeps prostate growth under control;
Nourish urinary and reproduction systems;
Stimulate sperm production;
Improve libido;
Provide better erections;
Retard hair loss and grow new and more hair;
Stimulate alertness and aggressiveness;
Re-activate the telomerase genes to slow aging;
Increase life span.

Testosterone replacement therapy, HRT, can restore youthful maleness in men and youthful libido in both sexes. HPT, properly taken, can approach the effectiveness of HRT.

9) Testosterone and the Heart

Many practicing physicians have been taught that testosterone causes men to have more heart attacks earlier in life than do women. This is a myth that has been proven wrong.

Proof is obvious by studying the cardiovascular risk factors, which **increase** as testosterone **decreases:**

Cholesterol and triglycerides levels go up, leading to increased arterial plaque;
Coronary artery and major artery dilation diminish - hence vasoconstriction and greater risk of cardiac events;
Blood pressure rises;
Insulin output is increased, which leads to obesity, elevated blood pressure, adult onset diabetes, and increased cortisone output;

Central abdominal fat is increased; increased waist/hip ratio;
Estrogen levels are increased - associated with higher stroke and heart attack rates;
Increased lipoprotein A;
Increased fibrinogen – the basis of most blood clots (combined with a simultaneous drop in Plasminogen, our natural clot buster);
Decreased human growth hormone (HGH) output, leading to a decline in energy, strength, stamina, and heart muscle mass and output;
Decreased energy and strength, causing decreased physical activity thereby leading to obesity ant the vicious cycle of the male Andropause.

**Low testosterone levels correlate with more
risk factors for heart disease
than does any other single factor.**

Testosterone level is far more important to heart disease than is cholesterol.

It is only a very small number of men that get heart disease without first showing some of the risk factors listed above: without first having low testosterone levels.

Testosterone is the heart-protective hormone of the male body - and it can be used to protect men from their major killer - heart disease.

And, for men that already have heart disease, testosterone can rescue them from its clutches.

The heart has more testosterone receptors than any other muscle. **The heart is the major muscular target for testosterone.** The heart's pumping power decreases when testosterone decreases.

Angina pains begin when nitric oxide production decline. Nitric oxide provides a function not unlike Nitroglycerine given to heart patients. Studies show that testosterone stimulates nitric oxide, which not only promotes erectile function in men, for which it is best known, but also promotes cardiovascular health in both sexes.

Nitric oxide is a neurotransmitter that stimulates the nerves causing male erection and vasodilatation; i.e. relaxation and improved blood flow in **all** major blood vessels including the Aorta - certainly not just the blood vessels supplying blood for erections.

In a test conducted by Dr. Shippen on an 80 year old with heart problems, high blood pressure, angina, and a history of transient ischemic attacks (TIA's), testosterone replacement cured his problems in less than four months. In six months he had resumed significant sex. In three and a half years his cholesterol has gone from 243 to 207 and his HDL from 41 to 55. He has had no further angina or TIAs. 80 years old!

In a test by Dr. Gerald Phillips at Columbia University College of Physicians and Surgeons, 55 males with chest pain or abnormal stress tests were evaluated. The findings were that the ones with higher testosterone had less advanced coronary artery disease and lower risk factors for fibrinogen and Plasminogen (the clot buster), insulin intolerance, and HDL was higher.

In the Caerphilly Heart Disease study of 2512 men in Wales, it was found that the men with heart disease had lower testosterone, higher insulin, and less HDL.

In a test in China of 62 elderly males with angina, testosterone was given to half and a placebo to the other half. 77% of those receiving testosterone had marked relief from angina compared to 6% for those taking the placebo. This indicates that blood flow to the heart improved 68.8% for those taking testosterone.

In a test by Dr. Shippen, testosterone replacement via a pellet in the buttocks effected the following changes:

At Start of Tests:		5 Months Later
Age:	49	
Height:	5'9	
Weight:	230	220
BP.	192/118	160/100
Cholesterol:	335	235
Triglycerides:	900	357
Blood Sugar:	192	140
Insulin:	70	15
Testosterone:	410	767
Energy:	Always Tired	Energetic
Sex:	Just OK	Very Good
Interest Level	Down	Up

When testosterone levels are low, the risk factors for heart disease are usually high. When testosterone HRT is administered, most of the major risks for heart disease diminish. HPT has a similar effect, although not as effective as HRT.

Testosterone replacement is vital for recovery of cardiovascular functions.

10) Testosterone and the Bones

The basic processes of bone build-up and re-absorption were discussed earlier, and it was explained that an osteoblastic stimulator is needed to create a sufficient quantity of Osteoblasts to rebuild the bone lost to re-absorption and other factors.

Testosterone and HGH are nature's best osteoblastic stimulators.

In a test in 1979, a 30-year-old man that suffered severe back pain was found to be in the early stages of osteoporosis. When tested, it was found that his testosterone level was a low 374. After receiving testosterone HRT for only two weeks, his pain ceased. Subsequent tests showed that his "new level of testosterone" had stimulated his rate of bone mineralization to triple.

Testosterone HRT for men, in some cases, can be far superior to HGH HRT alone for some bone disorders.

Women also frequently need testosterone HRT for certain, actually most, bone disorders. Testosterone can inhibit interleukin-6 (IL-6), which is a hormone-like substance that stimulates the cells in bone marrow. When IL-6 becomes too high, there are more Osteoclasts (the demolition cells previously described) than Osteoblasts. Therefore bone is destroyed faster than it is rebuilt.

So, bone mass and density decrease with age - as testosterone decreases with age. **Testosterone HRT and HPT stimulate** the body to re-build bone faster than it is destroyed so that the bone mass and density can **return towards youthful values.**

11) Testosterone and Sexual Function

As has been stated, testosterone is the primary sex hormone for men and is the hormone that drives libido in both men and women.

It is very interesting that sexual function and heart conditions in men are closely related. A decrease in sexual function almost always forecasts heart disease - and often - diabetes. These are conditions that are common to male Andropause.

Testosterone replacement is vital for restoring libido and sexual function for both males and females.

12) Adverse Side Effects of Testosterone HRT

Un-pure and/or synthetic testosterone can cause many side effects including liver damage. HRT must use only pure, natural, testosterone.

We must also make sure that the nutracuetials used in HPT are of high quality.

Even with pure, natural testosterone, there can be adverse side effects which **have been reputed** to include an increased risk for prostate cancer, atrophying of the testicles, high red blood cell count, depression, fluid retention, reduced sperm count and volume of semen, and a reduction in HDL cholesterol (the good kind).

Of all these concerns, the major concern with testosterone therapy for men has been its potential to stimulate and/or accelerate the growth of benign or malignant prostate tumors. The second major concern has been its reduction of the good HDL, which increases the risk of coronary artery disease.

A series of tests, as described in the next section, and more recent tests reported by Dr. Chein suggest that **neither of these concerns is warranted.**

According to Dr. Chein, it appears that testosterone HRT has no effect to increase prostate cancer. His tests show that testosterone replacement therapy lowers both the good and bad cholesterol.

Lowering the bad cholesterol may do more good than the bad done by lowering the good cholesterol.

Dr. Chein has stated that he believes this to be true and that the overall effect of lowering cholesterol with testosterone replacement therapy is an advantage.

Dr. Chein seems certain, but we still have a concern that men susceptible to prostate cancer should be weary of HRT and if they insist on using testosterone HRT should consider individually tailored dose levels and frequent blood testing.

We believe that HPT is a safer way to increase the availability of testosterone.

The third major concern with taking HRT is that the therapy can inhibit the body's own natural production of testosterone. If this happens, the patient must stay on the therapy for the rest of his life.

HPT avoids this potential problem in that it stimulates the body to use its own natural production system for testosterone.

These concerns simply mean that one must take great care when implementing testosterone replacement therapy. When taken in the proper dose, *tailored to the individual,* and when taken with DHEA *and the proper mix of the other enzymes and hormones,* and when alternating with Hormone Precursor Therapy, testosterone therapy can help turn back the clock on aging - and it can be safe.

HPT avoids the potential dangers and still provides most of the benefits of HRT. However it requires more time.

A special note for women; their risks are somewhat different because women naturally only have a very small amount of testosterone. It doesn't take a great deal to replace it to its physiologic levels.

When women take only small doses of testosterone there appear to be virtually no side effects. However, if the dose is too high, women can develop acne and unwanted hair growth on the body.

We need to make sure that we only put back the levels of that which has been lost with age. (See more details below at Adverse Side Effects of Testosterone HRT for Women.)

13) Testosterone and Prostate Cancer

Prostate cancer is the second most fatal cancer in American men (lung cancer is first). About 40,000 men die each year of prostate cancer.

Many physicians were taught, and thus still believe, that prostate cancer is caused by testosterone. The evidence indicates that this is not true.

Dr. A. Moogentaler proved, and published his findings in the Journal of the *American Medical Association* in 1995, that prostate cancer is associated with **low** testosterone.

A study at John Hopkins on fifty men showed no relationship between prostate cancer and testosterone.

Dr. C. W. Lovell treated over 300 men in his Louisiana Clinic for a period exceeding thirteen years with testosterone pellets. There was never a single case of prostate cancer.

Dr. George Debled in France reports very low instances of prostate cancers during the twenty years he has given testosterone to more than 2,000 men.

Dr. Shippen in the US reports that his patients with enlarged prostates (BPH) - but no cancer, all improved when he increased their testosterone levels.

A study in Japan - again of BPH - not prostate cancer - showed that the least prostate enlargement correlated with the highest testosterone.

Conversely, the Japanese study showed that in the cases where the prostate had become enlarged, such cases were associated with *high levels of estrogen*.

In an American study of 320 New England men with BPH severe enough for surgery - compared with 320 men without BPH - it was shown that BPH was more likely in men with low testosterone - and high estrogen.

Prostate cancer becomes common in men over the age of 80. Autopsies show that over 30% of men that died from all causes past 80 years of age had prostate cancer.

Fortunately, there are a couple of tests to catch prostate cancer before it becomes life threatening. These two tests are termed PSA and DRE.

When the prostate experiences BPH or cancer, it secretes an antigen termed prostate specific antigen (PSA). Typically:

AGE	PSA
Young	Near 0
Mid-Age	0-4 ng/dl
Problem	
Non-cancer BPH	4-10
Possible Cancer	10+
Most Likely Cancer	20+

This test is fairly accurate, but the DRE exam is highly recommended if the PSA exceeds 4, and in any case for men over the age of 50. The DRE is a Digital Rectal Exam where the doctor feels the prostate with his finger.

Excessive size will normally prompt a biopsy to test for cancer.

It should also be noted that a good test for indications of prostate cancer might be an analysis of concentrations of testosterone and its more powerful derivative, dihydro-testosterone (DHT). Intriguing support for such a view is offered by several medical studies that show that patients with prostate cancer have lower levels of DHT than patients with normal prostates or with BPH. The most recent of these, published in the *British Journal of*

Urology, found, indeed, that the more advanced the cancer the lower the level of DHT. The researchers speculated that a low serum DHT in patients with malignantly transformed glands "may indicate a loss of biochemical differentiation of the tumor."

14) Testosterone to DHT Conversion

Inappropriate testosterone **HRT** can also cause another kind of problem. The body has two types of an enzyme named 5-Alpha Reductases. There is one in the skin that stimulates oiliness to activate and deactivate hair growth. The second type is mostly in the prostate and it converts testosterone to a more potent derivative called dihydro testosterone **(DHT).** **DHT** is required by the body to perform many functions.

A primary function is to strengthen the fibro muscular portion of the prostate gland. This is vital for male potency and erections. A problem is that too much **DHT** can cause too much of this growth, resulting in prostate enlargement **(BPH)** and cancer.

Too much **DHT** can also cause other problems. **DHT** is a major cause of male baldness.

Standard therapy attempts to inhibit the levels of 5 alpha Reductases so that less **DHT** is produced. The result frequently causes atrophy of the testosterone sensitive cells in the stoma, i.e. the fibro muscular portion of the prostate. And, this can result in impotency.

15) Testosterone - Estrogen Balance

Young men have testosterone to estrogen rations of 50 to 1. As men get older, these ratios decease to 20 to 1. And sometimes get as low as 7 to 1.

Too much estrogen in men results in a neutering effect. Too much estrogen can be even "more neutering" than too little testosterone.

Further, as estrogen increases in men, it causes a slow down in testosterone production - which makes the problem even more severe.

Estrogen begins to occupy the testosterone receptors in the hypothalamus of the brain - tricking it into thinking that it is testosterone. The brain, thinking there is plenty of testosterone -

does not order more testosterone - and so testosterone levels further decrease.

The man's energy diminishes - sex life falters.

Let's examine what causes this increasing estrogen.

An enzyme called aromatase is widely present in the body and converts a certain portion of testosterone to estrogen. This is a simple process because testosterone and estrogen are chemically quite similar.

This conversion process is necessary for the healthy functioning of estrogen-sensitive tissues in the man's body. Estrogen, for example, is powerfully beneficial to the male brain. Estrogen is vitally necessary for male brain functions.

Too little estrogen will neuter a man just as effectively as too little testosterone.

The window of optimum effectiveness of estrogen in the male body is very small. The control mechanism aspect of estrogen can easily get out of balance as we age. Illness, lifestyles, etc., can cause such an out-of-balance situation to occur earlier in life than might otherwise happen.

Such an out-of-balance occurrence may well be the major cause of earlier male Andropause, as previously described. Too much estrogen in the male can cause several harmful effects:

Increased Clotting
Narrowing Coronary Arteries
Increased Risk for Heart Attack

These effects of too much estrogen in men are almost opposite the effects estrogen has in women.

The most common causes of the increases of estrogen in males during their midlife are:

Age-related increases in aromatase activity
Alteration in liver function

Zinc deficiency
Obesity
Overuse of alcohol
Drug-induced estrogen imbalance
Ingestion of estrogen-enhancing food or environmental substances

Almost all of these problems are interrelated, and one frequently reinforces or is the outright cause of another. Nonetheless, it's probably useful to take a first look at them separately.

Aromatase activity. First, there is aging itself. As a man grows older, he produces larger quantities of aromatase, the testosterone converter. Consequently he tends to convert higher levels of estrogen. It may well be that being overweight is the main reason for this apparently age-related change. When this is the case, aromatase increase is controllable. When there are other causes, steps to minimize it can be taken.

Liver function. Alterations in liver function involve the important P450 system - a primary processing system that eliminates chemicals, hormones, drugs, and metabolic waste products from the body. Among its many duties is the task of excreting excess estrogen from the body. A wide variety of factors (including alcohol intake) can impair this system and tends to do so with age. In many individuals, this results in a gradual buildup of estrogen. In fact, the P450 system may be the most important factor in metabolic Andropause.

Zinc deficiency. Zinc status is critical. Since Zinc inhibits levels of aromatase, the testosterone-to-estrogen converter, declining zinc will adversely affect the testosterone-to-estrogen ratio. Inadequate levels of zinc are extremely common in the American diet, particularly among the elderly.

In addition, alcohol, drugs, and disease can significantly lower zinc levels. Zinc is also necessary for normal pituitary function, without which the proper hormonal signals will not be sent to the testicles to stimulate the production of testosterone.

There is an interesting circular relationship here. Not only is zinc important for testosterone, but also testosterone has been found to be necessary to maintain levels of zinc in the tissues.

Clearly in men whose zinc status is inadequate, the vicious cycle that becomes established must be broken into at some point through zinc supplementation.

Obesity. Next - whatever your sex - plumpness will tend to estrogenize you. Since fat cells contain aromatase, an increase in fat cell population will cause an increased in testosterone-to-estrogen conversion rate. Moreover, obesity has been clearly associated with lower testosterone levels at all ages. It's not surprising, therefore, that overweight men almost invariably show signs of an unfavorable testosterone/estrogen ratio.

Alcohol Use. Heavy alcohol intake also causes a dramatic rise in estrogen. Women, for instance, can increase their circulating estrogen levels threefold after just one drink. The rise in men is less dramatic but very significant nonetheless. Alcohol is closely related to two aspects of the problem we just discussed: it inhibits the P450 system, and it decreases zinc levels.

Heavy drinking in men has long been recognized as causing high estrogen levels with such related symptoms as spider veins, reddish coloration of the palms, gynecomastia (enlarged breasts), and even testicular atrophy. Increased sexual dysfunction is also common. Shakespeare noted that *"alcohol: increases the desire but decreases the performance,"* and there is every reason to believe that alcohol-induced estrogen rises are a significant part of that effect.

Drugs. Certain foods, environmental substances and a variety of prescription drugs have adverse effects. Perhaps the most common class of problem drugs is the diuretics. Millions of American men are taking these "water" pills to treat high blood pressure. Though the effects on blood pressure are certainly good in the short term, long-term use of diuretics actually lowers life expectancy. One of the ways it does this is by removing sizable quantities of zinc from the body. As noted earlier, this increases aromatase, and the long-term estrogen increases that result may cause more cardiovascular damage in men than the diuretics prevent. It is necessary to take fairly high doses of zinc (50 to 100 mg. daily) to reverse these effects.

Supplemental testosterone HRT can correct unhealthy testosterone to estrogen ratios. It is interesting to compare two of the many tests that have been conducted on this issue.

A 55-year-old man was given testosterone HRT via injections because his testosterone was low. The results:

At Start		A Few Days Later
Testosterone	460	840
Estrogen	20	60

Testosterone shot up to 1200 initially, and then stabilized within 24 hours to 840. The estrogen increase from 20 to 60 was far too large a change and could do more damage towards neutering the man than his initial low testosterone would have.

Testosterone injections are always dangerous, because they momentarily elevate testosterone too high above "natural" levels - causing estrogen to go too high. For this reason, most doctors prefer the use of creams, and sometimes the patch.

In another test of a 58 year old man where testosterone was given via a patch:

	At Start	A Few Days Later
Testosterone	365	520
Estrogen	52	58

This test also resulted in estrogen at too high a level; however, this man already had his estrogen at too high a level. He was given zinc and soy protein with the following results:

| Testosterone | 500 |
| Estrogen | 30 |

This is close to the testosterone HRT goals that are practiced by those who are experienced in this field.

16) Atrophy of the Testosterone System

A possible adverse side effect of testosterone HRT is that it may cause the natural system to further shut down. Testosterone HRT providers typically give chorionic ginadotrophin (CG) in conjunction with testosterone to stimulate the system to prevent atrophy.

Those experienced in the field try to avoid this approach as a general practice, reserving its use for special cases that really need it. CG use for most cases is usually counter to the disorder that is causing testosterone to be low in the first place.

There are three commonly recognized endocrine disorders that occur, generally with age to cause a man to have low testosterone levels. One cause is the male Andropause previously described. The other two are known as primary and secondary hypogonadism. Hypogonadism is a medical term signifying reduced activity of the sexual organs or gonads.

Primary hypogonadism occurs when the Leydig cells in the testicles lose their capacity to secrete testosterone at youthful or near youthful levels.

Secondary hypogonadism occurs when - even if the testicles are capable - the control glands in the brain do not order the testicles to produce.

In young, healthy males the system works as follows:

When the hypothalamus portion of the brain detects that the circulating blood levels of testosterone are low;

It sends brief bursts of a hormone called gonadotrophin releasing hormone (GnRH) to the pituitary gland;

GnRH stimulates the pituitary to secrete luteinizing hormone (LH) and follicle stimulating hormone (FSH) at about one hour intervals;

LH and FSH stimulate the Leydig cells in the testicles to manufacture testosterone.

One must run blood tests to analyze the levels of testosterone, GnRH, LH, and FSH to determine the cause of low testosterone: i.e., primary or secondary hypogonadism. Additional tests are then required to determine the cause of the problem. The following tables list the typical causes.

Primary Causes of Hypogonadism

Hemochromotosis
AIDS
Cancer
Chronic Disease
Rheumatoid arthritis
Renal failure
Cirrhosis of the liver
Chronic obstructive pulmonary disease
Drugs (cancer chemotherapy, immunosuppressants, etc.)
Radiation
Hormone or follicle-stimulating hormone
Alcohol
Prader-Willi Syndrome
Laurence-Moon-Biedi syndrome
Delayed puberty

Secondary Causes of Hypogonadism

Pituitary or hypothalamic tumor
Granulomatous disease
Infarction
Trauma
Vascular Defects
Hyperprolactinemia
Nutritional deficiency or starvation
Massive obesity
Glucocorticoid drugs
Kallman's syndrome
Isolated deficiency of luteinizing
Genetic disorder

Secondary hypogonadism is the more common cause of testosterone deficiency in middle-aged men. It is almost always treatable.

CG is very similar in molecular function to LH. Generally speaking, CG is entirely effective at jump-starting the quiescent testicles.

In a typical test case of a 52 year old whose testosterone was very low: 272 ng/dl and both his FSH and LH were also low, he was given CG. One month later his testosterone had soared to 1,114 - way too high. He had manic energy and was irritable.

His dose of CG was reduced from three times per week to two times per week and his testosterone went down to the 800's.

A little CG had indeed jump-started his system.

Primary hypogonadism and the male Andropause require direct testosterone HRT for the most effective results. HPT can help but not as quickly or effective.

17) Adverse Side Effects of Testosterone HRT and HPT for Women

Excessive doses of testosterone can cause growth of facial hair and, in extreme cases, a deepening of the voice. Fundamentally, however, there is no justification for a woman ever taking doses high enough to cause such problems. Testosterone is a natural part of a woman's body, and the small supplemental replacement doses normally used by experienced doctors simply brings her back into her normal range - the place where she was from puberty to menopause; the period in which, in all probability, she felt at her physical best.

When taken in the proper dose, *tailored to the individual,* and when taken with DHEA *and the proper mix of the other enzymes and hormones,* and when alternating with Hormone Precursor Therapy, testosterone therapy can help turn back the clock on aging - and it can be safe.

Testosterone therapy for a woman whose levels have been less than ideal is going to notice a resurgence of energy, very possibly an improvement in muscle tone and relief from aches and pains, an improvement in bladder problems, and, in almost all cases, an improvement in sexual desire and energy.

HPT can produce almost all of the benefits of HRT without any of the side effects. It will just not be as quick and effective as HRT.

18) Testosterone Levels

Testosterone levels vary widely among men. Peak levels usually occur between the ages of 13 and 20. Ideal peaks average about 1080 ng/dl and then begin to drop with age as shown below.

Age	Percent of Peak
0	0
2	1.8
4	35
5	56
10	91.2
13	100
20	100
30	66
40	45.6
60	18.4
80	3.5

Significant health and performance problems occur when testosterone is below 500 ng/dl or below about 46% of one's peak. This frequently begins to occur in the forties and almost always occurs by the fifties.

Testosterone levels for women are typically 10% to 8% that of men until after menopause when the levels may remain at 10% of the levels for men, but frequently drop to only 2%.

19) Testosterone Precursors

The only effective testosterone precursor is DHEA. The dose level is either 50 or 100 mg of DHEA dependent on results of blood level tests and age.

20 Testosterone Summary

Proper levels of testosterone are necessary for optimum health. The benefits are enormous. There are essentially no adverse side effects of our HPT program. Tests have shown that the recommended DHEA is an effective and, when taken properly, safe precursor that will return testosterone levels towards more youthful levels and will, at least partially, re-activate the telomerase genes and slow aging.

Chapter 3
Estrogen

Estrogen is the principal female hormone that makes a female a female. The ovaries produce it. Estrogen is the most powerful hormone in the female body. It builds up in young females and peaks shortly after puberty.

Estrogen is also produced and used in the male body. It is vital for brain function, as previously described.

Most all tissues in the human body – over 300 – are affected by estrogen. The effects vary from person to person depending on their individual genetic profiles.

After menopause, the female body undergoes major changes because of a significant decrease in estrogen. As an example, the average woman's body at age thirty is 35% fat. By the age of eighty, it is 53% fat.

Estrogen, like testosterone, is an anabolic steroid, though it's anabolic (muscle – building) effect is significantly weaker. Its effect on physical shape, on fat deposits around hips and breasts and thighs, is well known. It is also a powerful protector of bone, a guardian of female cardiovascular health, a promoter of thick, smooth skin, and of course, a crucial component in the proper: functioning of the female sex organs.

Nothing in medicine has been studied so intensively for so many years and through so many patient trials and investigations as estrogen replacement therapy. Over forty million women have participated in this multi-billion dollar business. Most participants now also use the other key female hormone, progesterone, along with estrogen. Some use progestin, which is a synthetic form of progesterone.

The average woman has almost forty years of life, from puberty to menopause, in which to enjoy the health-promoting benefits of estrogen. During that time she is remarkably resistant to illnesses and to aging changes. A young woman is mankind's healthiest member. Heart attacks and strokes barely exist for women during this part of their lives. Arthritis, and other health problems are rare, and her immune system function is at its best.

And then menopause. The woman loses most of her estrogen. She begins to accelerate towards catastrophe.

1) Menopause

Menopause typically begins between the ages of forty-five and fifty-five with the average age being about 51. It is an extreme physical and emotional transition for most women. Menopause is a result of hormonal changes that may occur gradually over several years or may be sudden.

The best way to describe the cause of menopause may be to start with an understanding of a hormone called follicle-stimulating hormone (FSH). This hormone, released by the pituitary gland, triggers the growth of follicles in the ovaries. The ovaries, in response, secrete the hormone estrogen.

As menopause approaches, the ovaries become less responsive to FSH so the pituitary gland produces more in an attempt to maintain estrogen levels. These hormonal changes result in an increasingly irregular menstrual cycle and variable ovulation.

The first sign of menopause for most women is a noticeable change in her menstrual cycle. Bleeding may occur more often or less than it previously had. The length of the menstrual period may become shorter with lighter bleeding, or longer with heavier bleeding. In short, the menstrual period becomes highly unpredictable. The periods may not occur for several months and then reappear. However, about 20% of women will experience no changes in the menstrual cycle until menstruation stops suddenly and completely.

A common symptom of menopause is hot flashes. The secretion of the large amounts of FSH by the pituitary gland causes these. This excessive FSH hormonal imbalance causes the blood vessels in the skin to dilate and constrict irregularly. This then causes the hot flashes, and the associated sweating and headaches. Stress, a hot environment, eating spicy food, or drinking coffee or alcohol can trigger hot flashes by additionally affecting change in the blood vessels. However, about 20% of women do not have hot flashes. But some have them for more than 20 years after menopause!

A very significant result of menopause is a thinning of the vaginal walls. This causes a loss of elasticity and a narrowing of the vagina. It frequently results in dryness with an itching sensation.

Doctors began prescribing various estrogen replacement therapies in the 1940s.

86% of post-menopausal women report a decline in their libido and their level of sexual activity. Although some part of this change is due to estrogenic deficiency resulting in vaginal atrophy, loss of energy, and increased depression, most of it is actually caused by a decline in androgens.

Overall a woman's levels of testosterone typically decline by over 50% in the years after menopause. Half of this decline is due to the complete shutdown of testosterone production in the ovaries. Equally important, however, are the adrenal glands declining production of two other important steroids: androstenedione and DHEA. These two hormones cannot replace testosterone's contribution to sex drive on their own, but a process in various cells throughout the body converts them to testostcronc. It is called peripheral conversion.

The problems caused by menopause are becoming more and more numerous as women continue to live long beyond the onset of menopause. It is estimated that, worldwide, this population of post menopause women will increase by 47 million per year!

We should not leave this section on Menopause without mentioning "surgical menopause". More than 10 million women in the United States and twice that amount globally have had their ovaries removed for various reasons.

The ever-increasing problems resulting after menopause have to be addressed – and treated.

The population of postmenopausal women is rapidly growing worldwide:

| 1990 | 467 Million |
| 2030 | 1,200 Million |

2) Estrogen HRT

Estrogen replacement has been offered since the 1950s and is the most widely used of all hormone replacement therapies. However, because of the recent findings of adverse side effects, many women have stopped their HRT, and many others have decided not to start.

The principal fear is that HRT increases the probability of breast cancer. But before we rush to conclusions, let's review the widely varying test data in terms of benefits and adverse side effects.

We will see that HRT is highly beneficial for most women and presents specific, measurable, adverse side effects only for some – not all – women.

3) Benefits of Estrogen HRT

Over forty million women in the USA have received estrogen HRT. Most take HRT for the reduction of menopausal symptoms including hot flushes, mood swings, lost of energy, lost of bone density, and lost or reduction of libido. A very large number of researchers have studied various groups of these women – at various times – and for varying time periods. They have reported a wide range of conflicting results.

In 1999, a panel was convened to reach a "consensus" on estrogen **HRT**. They concluded:

Estrogen **HRT** will decrease the risks of osteoporosis;
Estrogen's **HRT** benefits to the heart are not yet clear;
Estrogen **HRT** may provide increased protection against:

Colon Cancer;
Dementia.
"Not yet clear...may provide." Typical of committees: no useful output.

Then in 2002 the very scary results of the Women's Health Initiative were published. The study followed 16,608 women aged 50 to 79 with the average age being 63 at the beginning of the study. The study lasted for a period of 5.2 years. 8,506 of the women were on HRT and 8,102 were given a placebo. The reported findings:

Affect On:	Risk per 10,000 Women
Breast Cancer	Increased 8 more
Heart Disease	Increased 7 more
Stroke	Increased 8 more
Pulmonary embolism	Increased 8 more
Colorectal cancer	Decreased 6 fewer
Hip fracture	Decreased 5 fewer

The scare caused by these results has been greatly exaggerated. Looking closer, it was seen that the women in the 50 to 59 age range – who are the majority of women needing the HRT – enjoyed decreased risks for heart disease and stroke. Additionally, detailed study of the results indicated that it was the use of synthetic progestin by the women that caused the increased risk of breast cancer. Estrogen per se – in other tests – reduced the risk of breast cancer, especially so when taken with natural progesterone.

We have carefully analyzed the various tests and studies – have taken into account the varying parameters: estrogen alone, estrogen with progestin, estrogen with progesterone, dose size, length of their HRT, the varying genetic profiles and the varying ages of the participants, and concluded that the benefits and adverse side effects are dependent on the health and genetic profiles of the individual, and on the combination, balance, and dose size of the HRT hormones. The combined results from all tests – other than the tests using synthetic progesterone, which should never have been used in the first place – show:

A decrease in heart disease that varies from very little for some women, to 60% for others;
A decrease in strokes that varies from slight to 75%;
Improved mental ability:
> Concentration;
> Alertness;
> Memory improved by 39%;

Retards:
> Dementia, and
> Alzheimer's disease from slight for some and up to 50% for others;

Reduces joint and muscle pain;
Retards onset of – and sometimes reverses – osteoporosis;
Keeps bones strong;
Keeps teeth strong – 36% less likely to need false teeth.
Reduces colon cancer by 29%; that increases to 55% when used for over 10 years;
Provides a slight decrease in lung cancer;
When taken with progesterone, the risks of uterine or breast cancer that may result from taking estrogen alone, are nullified;
Retards onset of cataracts;
Increases youthful qualities of skin: thickness, tone, etc.;
Relief from hot flashes, and other symptoms of menopause;
Improved mood;
Better sleep;
More energy;
Better quality of life;
Longer life: a 44% decrease in mortality over a given period of time.

Extends sex life:
> Improves libido,
> Decreases vaginal dryness,
> Improves vaginal wall thickness,
> Makes vagina more flexible,

Reverses vaginal atrophy.

This may seem to be an unbelievable list of benefits. But estrogen is the most powerful hormone in the female body.

Let's look at some more details.

4) Estrogen and the Heart

Many women simply are not aware of the fact that heart disease is the biggest single killer of women as well as men. In fact, all the evidence shows that if it weren't for the protection afforded them by their hormones; women would be significantly more at risk for heart attack and strokes than their male counterparts. Men have significantly large arteries, which take a lot longer to get totally blocked. Men are protected to a very large degree by their testosterone, but their protection does not compare with the protection that the female hormones give to women.

Once postmenopausal women lose their hormonal protection, they demonstrate a startling and dismaying ability to overtake the other sex; in less than fifteen years, they're having heart attacks as fast as men. Yet, in women who replace estrogen, this change does not occur.

The best estimates by reputable medical epidemiologists of estrogen's protective powers are simply stunning. One group of researchers reporting in the *New England Journal of Medicine* on 5,000 women on estrogen concluded, based on the improvements in their risk factors, that they would experience a reduction in their rate of heart disease of 42 percent. British researchers, analyzing their own data, came up with a figure of 50 percent.

It is not surprising, for there is hardly a single risk factor for heart disease in women that is not radically improved when a postmenopausal woman replaces estrogen.

Estrogen helps to lower Homocysteine levels and, in combination with vitamin therapy, will almost certainly have a significant life-saving effect.

The meaning of all these alterations in the cardiovascular milieu is best described by looking at each of these factors separately.

Cholesterol: As virtually every American is by now aware, cholesterol has something to do with heart disease. Its importance has been overstressed, but nonetheless, it is quite real. **LDL** cholesterol – the so-called " bad " cholesterol only causes problems when it has been oxidized by free radicals, the process that antioxidant vitamins like C and E help to protect against.

Once oxidized, however, **LDL** certainly is a bad player. Increased levels of it in the bloodstream trigger the activity of macrophages which are large cells that engulf bacteria and various unwanted debris, including the particles of **LDL** cholesterol. The engorged macrophages then become foam cells, and these trigger changes in the wall of the artery leading to plaque formation. Plaque then fills up and eventually entirely blocks the artery, the whole process being called atherosclerosis.

HDL cholesterol is called good cholesterol because it actually transports **LDL** out of the tissues and back to the liver for excretion. Estrogen's marked capacity to lower **LDL** cholesterol and raise **HDL** cholesterol is an important part of its cardiovascular protection.

Fibrinogen: This natural clot – forming substance in the bloodstream has been associated at high levels with a three – to five fold increase in the atherogenicity of LDL cholesterol. High levels of fibrinogen make it far more likely that a blockage in a major artery will result in heart attack. Estrogen is clearly associated with lower fibrinogen levels.

PAI-l: Plasminogen activator inhibitor (**PAI-l**) decreases the body's ability to inhibit the formation of blood clots and so increases the likelihood that complete blockage of an artery will precipitate a heart attack. Estrogen clearly lowers levels of **PAI-l.**

Homocysteine: Homocysteine is the newest buzz word in cardiovascular circles.

It derives from metqionine, an essential amino acid that is present at fairly high levels in the American diet. Adequate quantities of vitamins B-6, B-12 and folic acid break down Homocysteine, defusing its potential for harm.

Insulin and Glucose: Both insulin and glucose have been found at higher than normal levels – to correlate strongly not only with risk of diabetes but with risk of heart disease. A rise in insulin levels is so common that many doctor regard it as almost a normal, even if unfortunate, part of human aging. Estrogen's tendency to lower these risk factors may be highly significant in the over all cardiovascular protection it offers.

Lipoprotein (a): Levels of lipoprotein (a), a type of cholesterol that has particularly high association with risk for heart attack, seem to be largely determined genetically, but like testosterone, estrogen has turned out to be one of the few things that can effectively lower it.

Results vary from test to test – done at different times – by different researchers – with different groups of women. But it seems very clear that estrogen HRT will reduce heart disease by at least 40%.

These same factors that provide less plaque, better dilating coronaries, decreased clotting factors, and the revving up of the body's natural clot busting system also decreases the probability of strokes. Tests have shown that estrogen HRT will decrease strokes by 75%.

Caution: It should be noted that a very recent test suggests that these cardiovascular benefits of estrogen HRT may not be as great as the previous test have shown. This latest test, however, is very suspect because it is counter to the very large number of previous tests – and it was sponsored by NIH.

Dr. Bruce Ettinger and his associates studied nearly five hundred women who belonged to the Kaiser Permanente health system in California. Two hundred and thirty two of these women had been on estrogen replacement therapy for an average of seventeen years. They were compared with 222 women who had been on estrogen for an average of less than one year during the same period.

It was discovered that the death rate from all causes – for women on estrogen HRT – was lower by 44% over the time period studied.

The American Heart Association has taken the following position: "Since heart disease and stroke kill far more women than any other disease in this country (about one in two women die from cardiovascular disease), the American Heart Association is interested in any research that improves our understanding of how women's risk of cardiovascular disease can be reduced."

The American Heart Association emphasizes the following points:

The analysis report showed that in all women studied, hormone replacement therapy **reduced the risk of death from cardiovascular disease, as well as from all causes;**

While reduction of risk declined after ten years of treatment, there is still a positive effect – i.e., **a reduction in risk continues or persists** [even though it is declining] **after ten years;**

Each woman after menopause should talk with her doctor about what she can do to reduce her risk for cardiovascular disease. This includes: being physically active, following a healthful diet and not smoking. And, when the doctor and the patient agree, using post-menopausal hormone replacement therapy along with drugs to control elevated cholesterol and high blood pressure.

Women who take estrogen HRT experience improvement in almost all heart disease risk factors:

Higher levels of " good" HDL cholesterol
Lower levels of " bad" LDL cholesterol
Lower levels of fibrinogen
Lower levels of Plasminogen activator inhibitor (PAI-l)
Lower levels of Homocysteine
Lower levels of insulin

Lower levels of glucose
Lower levels of lipoprotein
Increases blood flow to all parts of the body, including the brain, heart, muscles, skin and bones – and sexual areas.

It is very clear that estrogen HRT, properly prescribed, and in proper combinations with other supplements, will almost certainly provide better heart health for women that have reduced hormone levels.

5) Estrogen and the Brain

Estrogen is vital for brain function. It helps provide the densest possible web of dendrites and axons, the neuronal filaments. These elements connect one brain cell to the next to improve communications. Estrogen accomplishes this by causing the brain cells to be more sensitive to nerve growth factor, a protein whose main function is to stimulate the growth of the dendrites and axons.

Moreover, a fall in estrogen triggers a decrease in blood flow to all parts of the body including the brain, heart, muscles, skin, and bone. Brain scans of the vascular system of the brain have showed increased circulation when estrogen is added. That means as well that there must be an increase in the delivery of oxygen and essential nutrients. It is difficult to overemphasize how important it is to keep the highways open.

Another benefit of estrogen HRT is its effect on enzymatic changes. Dr. Bruce McEwen, a neurobiologist at Rockefeller University in New York, has shown estrogen spurs the production of choline acetyltransferase, a major enzyme in the brain that is needed to synthesize acetylcholine. Acetylcholine is one of the brain's primary neurotransmitters, a substance that makes possible the final transmission of messages from one brain cell to the next.

People affected with Alzheimer's disease – the most damaging and irreversible of the dementias – have levels of choline acetyltransferase 60 to 90 percent below the human norm. For women, this is caused by a shortage of estrogen. There is no comparable male decline.

The brain is so richly supplied with the aromatase enzyme that by conversion from testosterone, a man's brain is kept richly saturated with estrogen, in sharp contrast with the relative estrogen deprivation a woman's brain experiences once her ovaries have shut down. Of course, on the male side, this depends on maintenance of adequate testosterone. When testosterone levels in elderly men decline too steeply, either because of natural changes or because of medical treatment that blocks testosterone, brain functions begins to slide downhill quite quickly and consistently.

This finding stimulates the question: "Will administering estrogen HRT to a postmenopausal woman prevent Alzheimer's? The answer is maybe – and is expected to become yes when more tests are completed.

Let's look at some more results.

In one of the more interesting tests of women with Alzheimer's disease, the test **subjects experienced some memory return after only 3 weeks of therapy!**

Additional evidence of such improvements comes from a study of 2,418 women over an eleven-year period. The women on estrogen in this test were 40% less likely to get Alzheimer's disease than the women not on estrogen HRT.

In another test, researchers at the University of Southern California studied 235 older women. Eighteen percent of those who had not had estrogen therapy were eventually diagnosed with Alzheimer's disease, compared with only seven percent of the women that had received postmenopausal estrogen replacement therapy.

In another, larger study, Dr. Victor Henderson of the University of Southern California examined the death certificates and medical charts of 2,529 women who had lived in leisure world retirement communities in southern California and who had died between 1981 and 1992. Dr. Henderson discovered that the women who had been on hormone replacement had been forty percent less likely to develop Alzheimer's disease. Moreover, the protection increased with length of use. Women who had taken estrogen for more than seven years were 50 percent less at risk.

A later study in New York City confirmed the pattern.

Doctors at Stanford University gave tests to seventy-two older women who were estrogen users for an average duration of thirteen years, and a control group of seventy-two women of similar age and education who did not take the hormone. It was discovered that the ability to remember names was 39 percent better among those on HRT.

Dr. Frederick Naftolin, chairman of the department of obstetrics and gynecology at Yale University School of Medicine stated the reason for such great benefits of estrogen HRT: "There is not a cell in the brain that is not **estrogen sensitive directly.**"

Dr. Rowe noted that by the age of eighty, one of six women has contracted Alzheimer's. It appears that estrogen replacement therapy could cut that number by half.

"We know now that women taking estrogen after menopause reduce their chances of getting cognitive impairments."

Dr. John Rowe, President
Mt. Sinai School of Medicine
New York.

The female body approaches disaster when it loses its most important hormone. Her brain cannot function properly without estrogen. The evidence is overwhelming:

Estrogen stimulates brain function and offers substantial protection against the worst of brain diseases.

6) Estrogen and the Bones

One of the most visible – and catastrophic – results of the lost of estrogen is the subsequent lose of bone. When we see the arms and legs becoming frail and the back beginning to stoop we realize just how important estrogen is to bone health. Let's discuss how this all works.

Osteoclasts are present throughout our lives. They continually break down the bone for it to be reabsorbed into the blood stream. Their counterparts are the Osteoblasts, which continuously build up the bones.

When we are young, the Osteoblasts dominate. During most of our adult lives they are in balance.

Estrogen works by reducing the Osteoclasts, and thereby preventing the increase in bone re-sorption that occurs following the onset of menopause. Estrogen does not seem to have any effect on increasing the rate of bone formation; it just slows its loss.

Progesterone, the other principal female hormone is, however a powerful bone-building hormone.

Testosterone is the other hormone that greatly affects bone health. A newer study has shown that the lower a postmenopausal woman's testosterone levels were, the greater her loss of height. This loss is a direct result of bone loss in the spine.

It is now clear that proper HRT with the proper mix of hormones and calcium and other supplements can stop – and in some cases – reverse bone loss.

7) Estrogen and the Skin

The soft, smooth, and attractive skin of a young woman usually changes dramatically after menopause. The wrinkling and coarsening of skin that comes with menopause is largely the result of hormonal changes. Studies show that the condition of a woman's skin depends more on the age at which menopause occurs than on her chronological age. Skin "age" is determined by how many years a woman goes without adequate estrogen.

Estrogen keeps the layer of subcutaneous fat under the epidermis firm and resilient. Estrogen maintains moisture in the skin by enhancing the production of hyaluronic acid, a substance that keeps water in the tissues. And estrogen maintains the thickness of the skin by supporting the production of collagen, the connective tissue that provides the structure and tone of the skin. When collagen production falls off as a result of estrogen deficiency, a woman's features quickly begin to sag. Reduced collagen, together with the loss of subcutaneous fat causes tissue to weaken and bruise at the slightest bump.

Researchers at King's College Hospital in London report that skin in women nearing sixty who do not take estrogen is only half as thick as the skin of women who do take estrogen HRT.

8) Estrogen and Sexual Function

Estrogen is the principal female hormone that makes a female a female. Nature created the female primarily to provide children to carry on the species of mankind. She is therefore empowered with one of nature's strongest hormones – estrogen – to enable her to do this.

Estrogen makes a young woman the healthiest member of our species, until menopause.

Nature did not really design her to live beyond menopause. But advanced hygiene and advanced nutrition, and advanced medicines cause women to live 30 years or so beyond menopause.

After menopause – after the female has given birth to her children and her fertility period is over – nature needs her to live only long enough to raise her last child. Her death after that is not significant to nature. And so our genes had no reason to design her to live longer.

Now women must consider the use of the same knowledge of advanced medicine [that gave her 30 years of life after menopause] to restore the hormones that menopause took away.

9) Adverse Side Effects of Estrogen HRT

But there are adverse side effects to HRT – and **they differ for each individual**.

Early tests, conducted in the 1970's indicated that estrogen **HRT** could increase the risk for breast cancer by 30 to 40% when taken for over 5 years. The tests indicated that the risk for ovarian cancer increased 40% when estrogen **HRT** was taken for 6 years, and 70% when taken over 11 years.

Similar tests reported that HRT also increased the risk of uterine cancer. Other tests indicated a slightly increased risk of venous thrombosis.

Scary.

Later tests in 1980 then showed that these elevated risks are essentially eliminated by the co-administration of progestin, a synthetic form of progesterone. But this combination increased the risk for breast cancer when taken for more than 5 years!

Analysis of the tests also indicated that estrogen HRT decreased the risk of ovarian cancer when taken for less than ten years – but increased the risk when taken over ten years.

The earlier tests of estrogen **HRT** without progestin, showed a significant reduction of the risks for heart disease. But analysis of the later tests after progestin was used with estrogen **HRT** to nullify uterine cancer risk, it was learned that the progestin had nullified estrogen's benefits for heart disease.

Tests conducted even later show still better results with the co-administration of progesterone rather than it's synthetic.

But then more very scary results from the Women's Health Initiative were published in 2002. See the results as previously presented.

The scare caused by these results has been greatly exaggerated and have lead to major confusion. We try to work through the confusion in a later section.

But this confusion has resulted in only 20% of postmenopausal women using any form of estrogen **HRT**. And, of the 20% that do start, 80% of them quit within three years.

The adverse side effects can usually be prevented for most women by tailoring the correct dose size and hormonal balance – with other hormones – to each individual. This is better described in Section 13.

Meanwhile, let's look at the cancer issue more closely.

10) Estrogen and Cancer

Almost all women fear estrogen replacement therapy because of the breast cancer risk. It should be a major concern. Breast cancer is found in 211,000 women in the United States each year. 40,000 die from breast cancer each year. If a woman lives long enough, **one out of nine will gets breast cancer in her lifetime.**

However, the breast cancer studies that have been conducted for estrogen with progesterone actually show relatively little relationship between estrogen replacement and risk of breast cancer – and many studies report no relationship at all.

The risk of breast cancer is there with or without **proper** estrogen HRT.

The tests do indicate that some women will increase their risk of breast cancer by taking estrogen HRT. The indications are that risks for these women prone to breast cancer will have their risks increased by 0.15% - that is an increase risk of up to 15 more cases of breast cancer out of 10,000 women. [The scary tests results of the Women's Health Initiative, released in 2002 showed 8 more cases of breast cancer out of 10,000 women. The results are actually higher for women prone to breast cancer.]

The increase of risk by 0.15% seems to be a small risk compared with the statistically well-established fact that a woman on hormone replacement therapy is far more likely to live a longer and healthier life than those not taking HRT.

A Kaiser Permanente study done in California, over a given period of time in 1996, found that the death rate from all causes was reduced by 44 percent in post-menopausal women who took estrogen HRT.

This study and others like it make it difficult to understand the reasoning of physicians who reject hormone replacement and who even argue that menopause itself does not have a serious negative impact on women's health.

The fact is that the loss of hormones–in both men and women---is part of the process by which nature leads us to old age and death.

It is also interesting to note that when women who are on hormone replacement do get breast cancer, their death rate is markedly lower than it is among breast cancer sufferers who never used hormones. This is because organs such as the breast and prostate stay healthy in the presence of adequate levels of estrogen and testosterone respectively. These hormones cause the typical breast cancers to be less deadly because of a characteristic of normal cells called differentiation.

Differentiation is the processes by which cells that have not yet taken on any particular function, differentiates to do their special assignment, i.e. to become a skin cell, a bone cell, or a breast cell, etc. Cancer causes the cells that became cancerous to lose differentiation. Cancer takes over cells and converts them to its own purposes, and in the process robs the cells of their functional nature. Eventually the cancer cells lose all functional resemblance to other cells in the organ or tissue where they're found.

But in postmenopausal women on estrogen replacement who do contract breast cancer, their cancer cells are different. The cells remain much closer to the normal type of breast cell than do the cancer cells of women not on estrogen HRT. As a result, the tumor is generally less advanced and tends not to grow as swiftly and aggressively as does a normal cancer cell.

Estrogen's processes of differentiation serves the women well because the differentiation process prevents the cancerous cells from becoming as severe as they otherwise would.

It should be noted that various pharmaceutical companies are now testing drugs that are expected to reduce the risk of breast cancer.

As for colon cancer, tests have shown that estrogen therapy will reduce this cancer by 29%. When estrogen was taken over a ten year period, the reduction increased **to 55%**

It should be noted however, that even if the risks of cancer of the uterus were not increased, estrogen HRT would most likely cause a slight increase in benign fibroid tumors in the uterus. It is also likely to slightly increase the risks for blood clots, gallstones, migraine headaches, breast tenderness, and weight gain.

Studies show however, that the probabilities of these adverse side effects occurring for an individual are less than one percent.

Such risks should be weighted against the substantial benefits described above.

11) Adverse Side Effects of Estrogen: Summary

The more conservative position is that estrogen HRT – even with progesterone – may slightly increase the risk of breast cancer. It may also increase the risk for ovarian and uterus cancer.

Even if the risks of cancer of the uterus are not increased, estrogen HRT will most likely cause a slight increase in benign fibroid tumors in the uterus. It is also likely to slightly increase the risks for blood clots, gallstones; migraine headaches, breast tenderness, and weight gain.

There are unresolved questions on estrogen's affect on strokes.

Studies show that the probability of these adverse side effects is slight i.e. less than one percent. Such risks must be weighted against the substantial benefits previously described.

Such risks can be essentially eliminated by using HPT instead of HRT.

12) Estrogen Levels

Female production of estrogen begins at birth and increases to about 70% of its peak at puberty which typically occurs at about age 12. Estrogen levels then reaches the peak shortly thereafter.

Estrogen then cycles monthly until menopause which typically occurs between age 45 and 55. The most likely age of the start of menopause is 51.

After menopause estrogen rapidly decreases towards zero.

Estrogen levels are typically:

Phase	pmol/l
Pre-pubertal	12-57
Follicular Phase	29-525
Near end of menstrual cycle Phase	126-478
Postmenopausal	23-103

Estrogen levels for men are about 2% of their levels of testosterone until about age 50, and then typically increases to about 5% of their levels of testosterone until about age 70. After 70 estrogen levels become about 14% of their levels of testosterone.

13) Estrogen Precursors

The only effective estrogen precursors are DHEA and progesterone. Taken in doses of 50 to 100 mg per day, DHEA can stimulate for increased estrogen levels for pre-menopause women. Direct estrogen replacement must be used for post-menstrual women.

The DHEA doses must be limited to these values to prevent suppressing the body's natural ability to secrete DHEA. And, because DHEA can act as an oxidant and disrupt normal cell function, it must be taken with antioxidants previously described.

Progesterone, while a precursor of estrogen, cannot be used as such in HRT and HPT programs that are trying to avoid direct hormones i.e. that are using precursors to stimulate for natural hormone secretions.

DHEA is an exception because, while a hormone, it is also a natural precursor, and it is safe at doses fewer than 100 mg.

Chapter 4
Progesterone

While estrogen is the primary female hormone – the secondary female hormone, progesterone, is vital for principal female functions. It is also produced primarily in the ovaries. Progesterone begins to be produced at the beginning of puberty, and then cycles monthly. It declines to less than 10% of its peak after menopause.

Progesterone causes the lining of the uterus to thicken in preparation for pregnancy, and when pregnancy occurs, is essential for normal functioning and the healthy development of the baby. At the end of pregnancy, a fall in the level of progesterone helps initiate labor.

But progesterone should not just be considered a female hormone. It is not a sex hormone; it plays no part in the secondary sexual characteristics which develop at puberty.

It plays a major role in the bodies of both men and women. Progesterone levels should be optimized to maintain good health. Levels vary considerably in women, rarely in men.

Progesterone is the precursor to the two sex hormones estrogen and testosterone.

It is secreted primarily by the ovaries in females and the testes in men. Smaller amounts are produced by the adrenal glands, the brain and glial (nerve) cells.

There are no great quantitative differences between men and women except in a woman's, latter phase of the menstrual cycle. It's in this last phase of the monthly cycle that progesterone levels rise considerably above that found in the first half or follicular phase. It rises from as little as less than 1 ng/mL to 20 ng/mL.

It is the fluctuating progesterone levels, together with the rise and fall of estrogen, that result in changes of mood, sleep patterns, cravings/appetite, PMS etc.

It is the ratio between estrogen and progesterone that causes problems. If there is too much estrogen in relation to progesterone then the problems become more severe.

Estrogen is an excitatory hormone, causing cells to divide and multiply, including fat cells. It's implicated in inflammation, cancer, endometriosis, fibroids, PMS, migraines/headaches, cravings, incontinence, generalized aches and pains, flaking nails and weight gain.

Progesterone, on the other hand, is a calming hormone, reversing or preventing the above symptoms.

Progesterone and estrogen are the two hormones currently given in HRT for postmenopausal women. Originally estrogen was replaced alone, but doctors discovered this increased the risk of uterine cancer, and so progesterone was added.

Recently a major test was terminated because it showed that the combination of estrogen and a synthetic version of progesterone caused an increase in some adverse side effects, as are described above in the Estrogen Section.

1) Progesterone and Cancer:

Early studies of women on estrogen HRT indicated that it increased not only the risk for uterine cancer, but also increased the risk for breast cancer. Doctors therefore began to switch from estrogen alone to a combination of estrogen and progestrogestin – a synthetic form of progesterone.

Provera is a synthetic form of progesterone that was, and is still widely used. The synthetics were used because Progesterone had been too expensive.

Natural progesterone is now available at affordable prices, and therefore most medical professionals recommend against use any of the synthetics.

2) Synthetic Progesterone

A good reason not to use synthetics progesterone is demonstrated by the following typical case of a woman on Provera. She was fifty-eight, and for five or six years, since her menopause had been absolutely miserable. Her body felt sore, and her brain felt battered from a long battle with her nerves. Her sex life had shriveled. She had retired at fifty-five, thinking that maybe with more time and less work all would improve. And, nothing had.

She had acute anxiety, periodically acute depression, and was subject to panic attacks. All her problems had started at her change of life. There were mostly vaguely psychiatric. She had tried a wide variety of anti-anxiety and antidepressant drugs with little effect, but plenty of side effects. She summed up her feelings: "I feel my life is totally out of control, and there's absolutely noting I can do about it."

And yet, what seemed mental was purely hormonal. As soon as she switched from Provera, the synthetic progesterone she was taking, to natural progesterone, and started applying a modest amount of testosterone cream daily, her "mental" problems vanished and her original talkative, bubbly personality emerged. Her sex drive came back; her energy soared.

Some of her depression had no doubt been due to the synthetic progesterone, which affects many women that way, but the other effects were almost certainly the result of putting androgens back into a body that was being totally deprived. Tests had shown that her ovaries were totally shut down, and her adrenal glands were producing virtually no DHEA or testosterone.

The use of Progesterone with estrogen HRT provides all the benefits of estrogen HRT and nullifies the potential increased risk for cancer.

The use of pure progesterone as opposed to use of one of its less costly synthetics will prevent the side effects that some women have to the synthetics.

There is, however, still a concern that estrogen-progesterone HRT can produce adverse side effects if used for 4 years or more. These concerns, however, can be minimized by taking the proper doses tailored for the individual, and alternated with Hormone Precursor Therapy, and closely monitored for any adverse side effects.

3) Progesterone and the Bones

Estrogen prevents the increase in bone re-sorption that occurs following the onset of menopause. Estrogen appears, however, to have no effect on increasing the rate of bone formation, which means it's important to set it in place as a sort of metabolic shield against osteoporosis before the ravages of bone loss occur.

In contrast to the effects of estrogen, a great deal of evidence now suggests that progesterone, its partner in the management of the female reproductive cycle, is a powerful bone-building hormone. In effect, this means that two out of three post-menopausal women who still have an intact uterus, and who should be taking progesterone and estrogen to protect themselves from the greater risk of uterine cancer that estrogen replacement alone may cause, are actually lucky. The progesterone they take will not only negate (and, according to some studies, even reduce) any increased risk of cancer; it will add a powerful building block to their plan for bone preservation.

4) Adverse Side Effects of Progesterone HRT

There are no known adverse side effects of progesterone at any dosage. This is because overdoses do not suppress the body's own production. This is because progesterone stimulates for its own synthesis.

5) Progesterone Levels

Progesterone levels are about the same for both men and women except for the woman's menstrual and pregnancy periods.

Progesterone levels for women are generally as follows:

Pre-ovulation is less than 1 ng/mL

Mid menstrual cycle is 5 to 20 ng/mL
Pregnancy is 11.2-90.0 ng/mL early stage
And 48.4-425 ng/mL later stage
Postmenopausal is less than 1 ng/mL
Male levels are generally steady at less than 1 ng/mL.

6) Progesterone Precursors

DHEA is a precursor for progesterone. Progesterone is also its own precursor. Thus the precursors taken for estrogen are also the precursors for progesterone.

Chapter 5
Dehydroepiandrosterone (DHEA)

DHEA is a hormone produced primarily by the adrenal glands from cholesterol. It is called the "Mother Hormone" because it is converted by the body; on demand, into other hormones including:

Estrogen
Progesterone
Testosterone
Androstenedione

About half of the body's DHEA is produced in the adrenal cortex, with the rest coming from gonads, fat tissue and (notably) the brain. The steroid synthesis pathway is Cholesterol > Pregnenolone > DHEA > testosterone > estrogen.

DHEA is also the "Mother Hormone" because it provides great health and longevity benefits. It begins to be produced by the male at the age of seven, increases to its peak at about age twenty-five, and decreases to near zero in old age as depicted in the previous chart.

Female production is less than the male – and peaks near age twelve and decreases with age as also depicted in the chart.

DHEA is a hormone precursor produced naturally in the adrenals, brain and gonads. The decline of DHEA production with age results in low serum DHEA that contributes to many age related degenerative diseases.

DHEA is a 'master hormone' metabolized in the adrenals to make other hormones. Supplementing with DHEA has been shown to increase energy levels, vitality and a sense of well-being

Nearly every cell in the body has receptor sites for this unique hormone. DHEA levels in the blood can indicate the present – and future status – of certain diseases, including:
Cancer
Immune system functions;

Cardiovascular disease;

Memory disorders; and

Aging status; i.e. normal vs. advanced or slower aging.

The DHEA levels in an individual are the best hormonal indication of how that person is aging. The slower one loses their DHEA, as they grow older, the slower they age.

1) Benefits of DHEA HRT and HPT

A very large number of tests conducted by many researchers, over a long period of time have shown that DHEA can provide the following benefits:

1. Enhance the Immune System, stimulating T-cell production that fights invading germs, and producing protection against:
Cancer
Atherosclerotic: It lowers cholesterol
and reduces plaque by 50%;
Osteoporosis;
Lupus;
Herpes;
Hepatitis B;
Influenza;
Diphtheria; and
Tetanus.

2. Adds neurons to the brain that:
Improves memory;
Helps with learning disorders; and
Retards Alzheimer's disease.
3. Helps with weight control:
Raises Metabolism;
Decreases Appetite;
Decreases fat storage; and
Converts fat to lean muscle.

4. Provides youthful Health.

5. Prolongs Life.

DHEA has been shown to prolong life by preventing and/or controlling or curing many of the diseases associated with aging. It enhances the Immune System and protects against the diseases listed above.

It lowers blood cholesterol and stabilizes blood sugar levels. It assists in weight loss and in the conversion of fat to lean muscle mass.

It deserves being called "The Mother of all Hormones."

In a test by endocrinologist Samuel Yen, DHEA increased muscle in both men and women, and the men gained strength and lost fat. But the most noticeable effect was the way the drug made people feel.

In a previous study of thirty middle-aged people, Yen found that 82% of women and 67% of men scored higher on a series of tests measuring their ability to handle stress, their quality of sleep, and overall well being when they were on DHEA. Dr. Regelson, a leading oncologist states: "If you want to maintain a youthful level of health, then you have to be youthful physiologically and that means maintaining youthful levels of these (DHEA) hormones."

DHEA wakes up elderly immune systems and restores them to youthful levels of efficiency.

Dr. Daynes of Utah mixed DHEA with his vaccines and showed a great improvement against hepatitis B, Influenza, Diphtheria, and Tetanus, and he also reported that DHEA stimulates T- cell proliferation – to fight invading germs.

And, studies have shown DHEA to work against obesity by raising metabolism, decreasing appetite, and decreasing fat storage. It decreases fat storage by blocking the glucose -6- phosphate – dehydrogenises enzymes (G 6 p D). That blocks the body's ability to store and produce fat.

DHEA decreases appetite by stimulating the body to produce cholecy to kinin (CCK), the substance that signals our brain that we are "full."

In a study in 1988, five normal weight men were given a dose of 1600 mg of DHEA per day for twenty-eight days. Their average body fat was decreased by 31% and replaced with the exact same weight in lean muscle. Their LDL dropped by 7.5%, thus protecting against cardiovascular disease.

Replacing our youthful levels of DHEA positively affects each and all of these effects of aging. DHEA can prevent and/or help cure many of the diseases of aging. DHEA can make us younger.

2) Adverse Side Effects of DHEA HRT

But a word of caution: High doses of DHEA will suppress the body's natural ability to produce DHEA. If one allows this to happen, then one has to continue to take DHEA for the rest of their lives.

Too much DHEA can also act as an oxidant to disrupt normal cell function. These concerns can be avoided by taking the proper dose levels and by supplementing it with the proper levels of antioxidants.

Experts in the field generally limit the daily doses to between 25 and 150 mg (as compared to the 1600 mg given in the 1988 study previously discussed). The precise level is individualized for each patient by detail blood and other analysis. Further, the daily doses are broken down into at least 2 (4 for the higher) doses per day to minimize DHEA levels at any one point during the day.

And the DHEA is always given as part of the antioxidant, enzyme, and hormone "soup" tailored to each individual as mentioned earlier and as described in a later section.

3) DHEA Levels

DHEA levels decrease after age 7 as shown.

Age	Men*	Women*
0	0	0
7	64	26
12	81	58
25	100	52
78	2	2
120	0	0

* In percent of peak levels for men.

The peak for men varies greatly from person to person. It generally occurs at about age 25 at a value of 125 to 619 microgram per deci-liter.

4) DHEA Precursors

The principal precursor for DHEA is Pregnenolone. Pregnenolone, as previously described, will also act as a precursor for progesterone.

However precursors for DHEA are not needed because it is safe to take DHEA directly as part of your HPT.

Chapter 6
Melatonin

Melatonin is a natural hormone that exists in all living creatures. It was discovered in 1958. It is produced by the pineal gland from the amino acid Tryptophan and was earlier determined to be secreted by the pineal gland in our brain. We now know that it is also secreted by other endocrine glands as described below.

Melatonin is the most powerful regulator of the body's biological clock and the immune system. It has been termed "The Wonder Drug."

1) Melatonin as the Biological Clock

That portion of Melatonin that regulates our biological clock is secreted by our "Third eye", the pineal gland located near the center of the brain, between the eyes. In some of the more primitive animals – such as reptiles – it is literally a third eye in that it is a light sensitive organ covered by a shield of clear cartilage.

The pineal gland helps govern circadian rhythms, i.e. our biological rhythms that take place over a 24-hour day. In more primitive animals, it also governs seasonal cycles of mating, migration, and hibernation.

Tests have shown that when people spend fourteen hours or more a day in darkness that they return to primordial sleep patterns – during which they produce the high levels of Melatonin our ancestors experienced. And the return to the natural pattern of restful sleep.

But the levels of Melatonin decline as we age. As they decline, we get sleep problems such as insomnia. A Gallup survey reports that 49% of American adults – mostly older people – suffer from insomnia.

Dr. Steve Novil of the American longevity Research Institute has been treating patients with Melatonin since 1990 – and their insomnia has been cured.

Studies and tests by The University of Surrey in Britain, and by French researchers have shown that Melatonin can be used to "reset" our internal clock as a cure for jet-lag by taking 8 mg of Melatonin on the day of the flight and for three days thereafter, the test subjects were able to sleep better, focus better, and experienced fewer mood swings then did the control group that took a placebo rather than Melatonin.

2) Benefits of Melatonin HRT

But, Melatonin is much more than "a sleeping pill." Its benefits include:

Cure for insomnia
Resets "clock" from travel
Lethal to some Cancers:
Melanomas
Breast;
Prostate;
Inhibits others (but this is less proven);
Protects against chemotherapy induced toxicity;
Protects against a variety of degenerative and age – related neurological conditions of the brain, including:
Parkinson's disease
Alzheimer's disease
Schizophrenia; and
Depression;
Protects against other diseases including:
      Diabetes;
      Asthma;
      Down's Syndrome; possibly aids;
Protects against cataracts;
Lowers cholesterol;
Increases sexual interest;

Grows sexual organs back to youthful sizes;
Keeps thymus gland active into old age – further improving
immune system;
The very best antioxidant to fight free radicals;
Increase life span; and
Restores youth.

Dr. Walter Pierpaoli was the first to show that Melatonin treatments can extend the life span of mice by 25%. Others have increased this to 200%. These experiments were verified and extended by Dr. Pierpaoli working with Russian Dr. Lesikov. They transplanted the pineal glands from old mice to young mice, and vice, versa. The old mice lived out the longer remaining life spans of the young mice and vice versa.

Converting "mouse life" to human life, suggests that Melatonin treatments alone could increase human life span to 150 years. (Or at least 120 years – to the limits caused by telomere erosion previously discussed.)

One of the principal reasons Melatonin can extend life is that it is the very best natural scavenger of free radicals. It is nature's best antioxidant. It removes the free radicals (oxidants) from our cells. Otherwise they will cause cell damage – even DNA damage.

Studies have shown that Melatonin is a more powerful antioxidant than vitamins E and C for acting as a "free radical scavenger" and for protection against aging. Melatonin is also more efficient than vitamin E as a scavenger of the peroxyl radical, which contributes to massive lipid destruction in cell membranes.

Melatonin also protects against a variety of degenerative and age-related neurological conditions of the brain, such as Parkinson's disease, Alzheimer's disease, schizophrenia, and depression. Melatonin has also been shown to prevent cataracts.

Melatonin enhances the immune system and has been found to have a powerful inhibitory effect on some cancer cells. Further,

Melatonin has been shown to amplify immune effects of interleukin-2 and to protect against chemotherapy-induced toxicity. In tissue cultures, Melatonin has direct lethal action on melanoma cancer cells and estrogen-sensitive breast cancer cells. Melatonin has also been found to inhibit prostatic cancer cells from proliferation.

Also related to immunity is the research that has shown the dramatic effect of Melatonin on the thymus gland. The thymus gland is important in the defense against infection. The thymus gland undergoes a transformation as we age. The thymus gland grows steadily larger as we approach puberty, and then begins to shrink until, in old age, it has virtually disappeared. As the thymus declines, so does our infection-fighting ability. Melatonin appears to protect this gland and improve its function, as we grow older.

Tests have also shown that Melatonin may be effective in treating diabetes, asthma, cataracts, Down's syndrome, breast cancer, and even AIDS.

It appears to help with other cancers. Doctors in Milan added Melatonin to their chemotherapy and immunotherapy and got significant tumor reductions that enabled their cancer patients to live longer.

It was most effective in treatment of breast cancer, where it almost always retarded it, and frequently cured it. Early tests indicate that it may be equally effective against prostate cancer – a cancer chemically related to breast cancer.

It also lowers cholesterol – in those who have high cholesterol – thereby helping to prevent heart disease. It does not appear to affect cholesterol when cholesterol is at normal level.

These tests results suggest that – in humans – Melatonin has evolved to become a much more versatile hormone then it is in more primitive animals.

Dr. Pierpaoli believes that Melatonin has evolved to become the principal "messenger" that tells our bodies when to enter puberty and when to begin sexual development; when to start each menstrual cycle in females, when to put us to sleep, when to wake up, and when to produce antibodies to combat disease.

Dr. Klatz has likened the pineal gland to the orchestra conductor that uses Melatonin as a kind of baton.

It appears that as we evolved, and Melatonin took on all these messenger functions, that it also began to be produced in glands in addition to the pineal gland. Very recent studies have shown that Melatonin is also produced in the retina – which acts as a photo-protectant to light sensitivity in the eye. This probably evolved as our "third eye," the pineal gland, regressed back into the brain and could no longer directly sense light

The very recent studies have also shown that Melatonin is produced in the endocrine cells that live in the gut. In fact, it seems that the gut now produces more Melatonin than the pineal gland.

The authors speculate that as Melatonin took on ever increasing roles as messengers to various organs, that glands closer to the source of "messenger" developed. Thus the gut produces its own Melatonin as a messenger to the thymus – which plays a pivotal role in

Melatonin stimulates (gives the message to) the thymus to release the T-cells that fight invading germs.

Melatonin treatments have also rejuvenated patients' sexual interest and in several cases have caused sex organs to grow back to their youthful size.

In summary, Melatonin restores youth.

3) Future Benefits of Melatonin HRT

Melatonin is now being studied to develop treatments for (1) stress, (2) improving immune system, (3) helping with mental disorders, and (4) as an ingredient in a new birth control pill.

4) Adverse Side Effects of Melatonin HRT

All tests have shown that Melatonin is completely harmless to the body at all dose levels. High doses, however, can cause a natural drowsiness and therefore should be taken only at bed- time.

Experts in the field limit the amount and timing of Melatonin treatments. Proper doses simulate the amount and release cycles of the youthful body. Proper Melatonin therapy always uses Melatonin only in conjunction with the other elements of the enzyme/hormone "soup" as previously mentioned and as detailed in later sections.

5) Melatonin Levels

Melatonin levels are the same for men and women. It helps the body know when it's time to sleep or when it's time to wake up.

Melatonin is released at night or in the dark and sort of instructs the body that it is time to sleep.

Young and middle-aged adults usually produce about 5 to 25 micrograms of melatonin per night. This level declines as a person ages and this is reported to be the reason why older persons have difficulty sleeping.

The decline with age is as follows:

Age	Percent of Peak
0	70
3	100
10	59
15	29
20	16
30	9
80	4
120	0

6) Melatonin Precursors:

There is no need to take precursors for Melatonin because you can take Melatonin directly. Tests have shown Melatonin to be safe at all dose levels, except it will cause drowsiness at high doses. Therefore it is best to take Melatonin only at bedtime.

The best long term dose level is three mg at bedtime.

Chapter 7
Pregnenolone

Pregnenolone hormone is a steroid precursor produced in the brain and in the Adrenal gland. It is a precursor for DHEA and progesterone hormones – which are produced from Pregnenolone based on the body's need. DHEA and progesterone are then precursors for the specialized steroid hormones:

Cortisol
Aldosterone
Estrogen
Testosterone

"Of all the hormones in the body, the precursor hormone, Pregnenolone, may be the most important for health and longevity."

D. Gary Young

"If DHEA is the mother hormone, Pregnenolone is the grandmother, because it is the precursor to DHEA."

Dr. Chein

1) Early History

But most people have not heard about Pregnenolone and its amazing benefits. One reason has to do with drug companies and profits as described below.

Pregnenolone research in the early 1940s was very promising and showed that Pregnenolone is effective in relieving arthritis pain, reducing PMS and menopausal symptoms, fighting stress and fatigue, improving memory, and lifting mood. But just as this research was being printed in medical journals, the discovery of synthetic cortisone was announced.

Drug companies could patent their laboratory version of cortisone and then make huge profits.

Pregnenolone, however, is a natural substance and is not patentable. Because synthetic cortisone was so fast-acting and offered great profit potential, **Pregnenolone research was basically abandoned.**

It was not discovered until later that cortisone had terrifying side effects (immune system suppression and osteoporosis being the two most devastating).

Pregnenolone has been shown to be virtually free of side effects.

A man in one Pregnenolone study did develop a temporary rash; while in another study on memory, a participant reported the "side effect" of decreased symptoms of arthritis!

2) Pregnenolone and Arthritis

The beneficial effects of Pregnenolone on arthritis and other bone, joint, and muscle diseases are well documented. In two studies on ankylosing spondylitis-an inflammatory disease of the joints that causes back pain and stiffening-patients showed marked improvement when treated with Pregnenolone.

Tests have also shown it to be anti-inflammation. It was widely used to treat rheumatoid arthritis until the discovery of the more effective cortisone that is now used for this disease. It is still used for patients that cannot tolerate cortisone's adverse side effects.

Neurobiologist Dr. Eugene Roberts studied the arthritis research from the 1940s and 1950s and said: "Treatment with PREG (Pregnenolone) can be maintained indefinitely without apparent harmful effects and is much less expensive than with ACTH or cortisone or with other anti-inflammatory steroids."

In addition Pregnenolone provides other significant biological functions throughout the body and provides the benefits described below.

3) Pregnenolone and Memory

Pregnenolone has long been known as a "memory" hormone.

In a recent study Drs. John E. Morley, James F. Flood, and researcher Eugene Roberts studied the effects of several hormones on the learning and memory abilities of rats. Researchers taught the rats the route through a maze. Then the rats were given DHEA, Pregnenolone, or testosterone.

To test the effect of the hormones on memory, the rats ran the maze again one week later. The Pregnenolone-treated rats greatly outperformed even those that were given the other hormones, and this performance was achieved using unbelievably small doses of Pregnenolone.

Research on memory by Rahmawhati Sih, Ph.D., showed that after older men and women were given Pregnenolone, the memory tests given three hours later showed gender variation. The women rated higher in verbal recall, while men improved in visual spatial tasks that required three-dimensional thinking.

The dramatic results of this test and the earlier human tests from the 1940s earned Pregnenolone the title of most powerful memory enhancer, up to 100 times more powerful than other hormones.

4) Pregnenolone and Alzheimer's Disease

Positive discoveries have led to current studies, including several currently evaluating the potential of Pregnenolone to treat Alzheimer's disease. Many people believe Pregnenolone could be effective in treating even full-blown Alzheimer's disease, because studies have shown that Alzheimer's patients have much lower levels of the hormone than healthy individuals of a similar age. Pregnenolone may also aid in Alzheimer's treatment because it is a precursor to estrogen and progesterone which, in recent years, have been shown to help prevent the onset of this terrible disease.

5) Benefits of Pregnenolone HRT

Tests have also resulted in Pregnenolone being recommended for all diabetes over the age of 40, and sometimes even younger diabetics.

Pregnenolone can also be a great help for easing the trauma of menopause. This is especially true for the dreaded ordeal for the millions of women who choose not to use estrogen replacement therapy because of a four to eight time higher chance of uterine cancer.

Part of the reason Pregnenolone has such a powerful effect on so many areas of the body is its grandmotherly role. As Pregnenolone levels increase, typically so will those of DHEA and the sex hormones of which it is a precursor. This is part of what allows Pregnenolone to improve overall physical and mental health.

Recent studies have shown that male and female bodies use Pregnenolone differently. Given the same amounts of the hormone and the same tests, results vary by gender. The conclusion from these studies is that in women, more of the Pregnenolone becomes estrogen, while men use more Pregnenolone to make testosterone.

As the parent hormone from which all other vital steroid hormones are made, Pregnenolone has been intensively studied for its effects on health, longevity, and emotional well-being.

Pregnenolone is made from cholesterol in the body. In turn, it can be synthesized into a number of hormones – estrogen, progesterone, testosterone, DHEA, Aldosterone, cortisol, etc. It is, in fact, the master hormone from which all the steroid hormones are derived.

A rising tide of clinical research is just beginning to show the powerful therapeutic benefits of natural Pregnenolone. Benefits that can reverse decline, balance hormones, and increase longevity. All in a completely natural substance that is non-toxic and virtually without side effects!

You can rest assured that Pregnenolone is well tolerated and its safety has been well documented. William Regelson, M. D., and Carol Colman stated in their book, **The Super-Hormone Promise: Nature's Antidote to Aging.** "We know that

Pregnenolone is safe, well tolerated, and causes no know side effects..." he stated.

6) Some Concerns

The body needs the following components to produce adequate amounts of Pregnenolone:

Cholesterol
Thyroid hormone
Certain enzymes
Vitamin A

If levels of these components are insufficient, the Pregnenolone supply will be too low. This can result in obesity, memory impairment, and old age-related disorders.

7) Lack of Cholesterol Hurts Pregnenolone Levels

Now, scientists and researchers are again looking at the value of Pregnenolone. The research that D. Gary Young found establishes how Pregnenolone declines in the body more than 60 percent between the ages of 35 and 75. Along with this natural bodily decline, our bodies have had to deal with a decrease in the building block of Pregnenolone – cholesterol. "Low cholesterol" or "no cholesterol" has been pounded into the heads of health-conscious consumers.

While the cholesterol link to heart disease is under question today, cholesterol-lowering drugs are causing hormone imbalance. Without cholesterol, there is no Pregnenolone, which means the body cannot create the hormones it needs.

The lack of cholesterol (and thus Pregnenolone) in our diets may be the cause of many cases of depression. Dr. William Regelson writes that: "A recent study conducted by the National Institutes of Mental Health showed that people with clinical depression have lower than normal amounts of Pregnenolone in their cerebral spinal fluid (the fluid that bathes the brain)."

Spinal cord injuries may be minimized with Pregnenolone according to a number of rat studies. Dr. Eugene Roberts would like to see a Pregnenolone cream placed in first aid kits for use on the spine following earthquakes or accidents.

He explained the value of the Raindrop Technique where certain oils are dropped along the spine: "Along the spine happens to be one of the largest accumulations of receptor nerve sites, and that's why Raindrop Technique works so specifically. When the oils get in there and can start stimulating nerve transmission – that's very, very important. When you combine the oils with Pregnenolone, then the oils carry the Pregnenolone into the cell structure to start that cell's rejuvenation. It is win, win, win, and balance, balance, balance."

Men are also susceptible to the age-related loss of Pregnenolone in the body. They needn't fear that Pregnenolone might be turned into a female hormone.

8) Adverse Side Effects of Pregnenolone HRT

There are no known adverse side effects at any dosage. This is because overdoses do not suppress the body's own production. This is because Pregnenolone stimulates for its own synthesis.

So while Pregnenolone treatments per se appears to be completely safe, we need to monitor all the hormones to make sure that the use of Pregnenolone, acting as a precursor for other hormones, does not adversely affect them. We have already shown that too much DHEA, estrogen, or testosterone in the body can cause some unpleasant side effects. When your physician carefully monitors not only your Pregnenolone levels but all your hormone levels, you can safely enjoy the benefits of Pregnenolone including increased mental acuity, better memory, and a greater sense of well-being.

9) Pregnenolone Levels

The levels of Pregnenolone are about the same for both males and females. The levels are very high at birth: 109 micrograms per deciliter of blood. During the first day of life, levels drops to about

86, and then further decrease to about 53 during the first month of life.

The decrease continues down to about 11 between the fourth and sixth month, and to about 3.7 between the seventh and twelfth month

Brain concentrations of Pregnenolone peak at around age thirty and decrease significantly thereafter.

1) Pregnenolone Precursors

Pregnenolone does not need any precursors. You can take Pregnenolone directly in 50 mg doses, two times per day.

Chapter 8
Thymus Hormones

The thymus gland which is located in the thorax behind the sternum (chest bone) secretes thymus hormones. It is the primary lymphatic tissue that secretes thymus hormones. Its function is to secrete hormones to nurture lymphocytes.

There are two types of lymphocytes: killer cells that destroy "foreign substances," i.e. bacteria, viruses, cancer cells, and other foreign bodies that are not a natural part of the healthy body; and helper cells that locate and mark the foreign substances for the killer cells.

The thymus provides at least six types of cells:

Interleukin 1 which is a class of proteins that are secreted mostly by macrophages and T cells.

Interleukin 2 is another version of the Interleukin proteins.

Interleukin 6 is yet another version of the Interleukin proteins.

Thymosin is a hormone that influences the development and differentiation of T-cells.

Thymopoietin, with the formal name of thymin is any one of three polypeptide hormones that result by alternative splicing of the same gene.

Thymulin is a zinc-dependent thymic hormone that regulates the differentiation of the immature thymocyte (precursor of a T cell) subpopulation and the function of mature T and natural killer cells.

The combination of the last 3 items is known as thymic humoral factor (THF), and is frequently used in HRT in place of the full set of thymus hormones.

The thymus gland is large at birth. It atrophies a great deal by age twenty.

The thymus hormone level builds to a peak at puberty, and goes to less than 20% of its peak by age twenty. It then continues to decrease linearly to less than 10% of its peak by age eighty.

The thymus gland is the major part of our immune system. In childhood this gland helps develop our immune system, with its principal task being the creation of T-lymphocytes, the specialized cells that find helper cell lymphocytes and eliminate bacteria, viruses, and foreign matter from the body. In late childhood, the thymus is the size of a plum, but at puberty it begins to shrink, and by the time we reach old age it is no larger than a small raisin.

Some of the functions of the thymus get transferred to other areas of the body such as the lymph nodes and bone marrow, but the atrophication of the thymus has a well-defined relation to immune system decline.

It's interesting that according to the statisticians, a human being is least likely to die of disease at the age of twelve, when his or her thymus is in full flower, than at any other time in life.

We now have considerable evidence in animals and some indications in humans that HGH could regenerate the thymus. Research in the 1980's on dogs showed that when growth hormones were inserted, "the thymuses of growth hormone-treated dogs regenerated, and resembled the thymic tissue of young dogs."

In 1991 David Khansari and Thomas Gustad of North Dakota State University completed a long-term study on mice. Taking fifty-two mice that had reached the age of senescence (approximately seventeen month,) they divided them into two equal sized groups with one group receiving growth hormone for thirteen weeks. Most of the members of that group were still living after all members of the control group had died.

Thymus function provides for the development of:

The killer and helper lymphocytes;
The central nervous system; and
The pituitary gland in the brain

The operative word for the thymus gland is "development." When a person's development is complete – by age twenty or there about – the gland's secretions decrease to the point that we cease to "develop" – and we then begin to age.

The deterioration of the thymus gland is closely linked to learning and memory abilities; and to the age-related diseases.

All six of the hormones that are secreted by the thymus gland are found to have an effect on T-lymphocyte differentiation and activation. The three hormones that make up the thymic humoral factor, i.e. Thymosin, Thymulin, and Thymopoietin inter blood circulation and act on the lymphocytes and tissues at various sites in the body.

1) Benefits of Thymus HRT

Research has identified the dependence of the central nervous system's development on thymus gland function. Other studies have established an important interaction between the thymus gland and the development of the pituitary gland in the brain. The age-related deterioration of learning and memory abilities has also been linked to the atrophy of the thymus gland.

In addition to the central nervous system, the thymus gland may also affect functions of other endocrine tissues. For example, congenital absence of the thymus gland is associated with alterations of the pituitary gland, adrenal gland, thyroid, and ovaries.

Anti-thyroid drugs that induce hypothyroidism also cause a marked atrophy of the thymus gland.

T-4 is one type of thyroid hormone. When its levels were reduced following anti-thyroid medication treatment, the thymocyte population in the thymus gland was also reduced. Conversely, when T-3, a different type of thyroid hormone, was administered in mice, multi-facilitated effects included increased weight and cell population as well as enhanced thymocyte production.

Within thirty days after surgery, removal of the pituitary gland resulted in a 50% reduction in both thymus gland weight and concentration of the thymus hormone known as Thymosin.

Over the past twenty years, at least four separate and distinct thymus preparations have been isolated and analyzed for T-lymphocyte regulating properties. Thymosin, Thymulin, Thymopoietin, and thymic humoral factor (THF) have been utilized as thymic hormonal preparations for hormone replacement therapy. Thymosin (TF) is a group of low molecular weight proteins extracted from bovine thymus.

Thymosin has displayed potent stimulatory effects on T-lymphocyte-mediated immunity. Thymosin increases lymphocyte activity and enhanced IL-6 production in spleen cells. Thymosin had a stimulating effect on luteinizing hormone and genadotropin releasing hormone, both pituitary hormones, in vivo studies of pituitary tissues.

In vitro Thymosin studies show that another pituitary hormone known as prolactin is released along with human growth hormone and adrenal corticotrophin (ACTH).

Thymosin is a protein extracted from porcine thymus tissue. It affects the differentiation of immature bone marrow cells and the function of T-lymphocytes.

This thymic hormone stimulates "killer cell" lymphocyte activity in the spleen cell cultures obtained from old, but not young, mice. The serum level of Thymulin decreases with age, and it coincides with thymus atrophy. Thymulin requires zinc for full biological activity.

Patients who suffer from Crohn's disease or acute lymphoblastic leukemia are zinc deficient. They also have a reduction in Thymulin activity. Young and old rats increased circulating Thymulin levels in response to administration of growth hormone and thyroid hormone injections.

THF is an extract of calf thymus. Interleukin-2 is a protein manufactured by lymphocytes. It was enhanced by the influence of THF in spleen cell cultures. Peripheral blood obtained from patients with chronic hepatitis B and viral infections responded to THF with increased production of IL-2. This suggests a possible antiviral role for this thymic hormone.

Thymopoietin is a protein isolated from bovine thymus gland. Thymopoietin enhances T-lymphocyte differentiation and effect of function on mature T-lymphocytes.

Various studies teach that the thymus gland and thymic hormones contribute to human immunity and to the neuroendocrine system. Additionally, alteration in the status of the thyroid, adrenal, and pituitary glands, as well as the kidney, have affected the structure and function of the thymus gland. Finally, results indicate that the presence of thymic hormone in circulation can have an affect on a variety of other organ systems.

Studies and tests have thus shown that thymus hormone replacement therapy tends to revitalize the body and contribute to more youthful performance of our various systems:

Immune system;
Neuroendocrine system;
Reproductive system;
Central nervous system;
Probably all other systems and glands (not well documented).

In summary, replacement of thymic hormone elements greatly enhances the immune system and tends to inhibit many age-related diseases.

2) Adverse Side Effects of Thymic HRT

There have been no adverse side effects noted.

3) Thymus Hormones Levels

The thymus hormones build until age 12 and then decrease significantly after age 20.

Age	Percent of Peak
0	0
1	1
2	3
5	30
10	95
12	100
14	95
20	18
22	16
24	15
40	10
80	8
129	0

4) Thymus Hormone Precursors

There are no effective thymus hormone precursors per se.

However some physicians have recently begun trying to rejuvenate the immune system by prescribing thymic hormones or peptides. What they've found is impressive.

Thymus is the peptide of tomorrow; it is on the horizon and poised to become a "super-hormone." We expect that we will soon be seeing articles and advertisements extolling the virtues of thymic supplements as frequently as we see those for DHEA or melatonin.

Because several of the thymic peptides are considered by the FDA to be dietary supplements, they are not regulated substances and are available for purchase at most health food stores. Others require a prescription.

You should be aware that, in order to get any benefit from the thymic peptides, you must have enough vitamins, minerals, and enzymes in your body. In fact, the thymic formula is inactive without these other ingredients. This means that you should take multivitamin supplements that include B complex vitamins, vitamins E and C, selenium, zinc, and beta-carotene. We also include various amino acids in the formulas.

Chapter 9
Thyroid Hormone

Thyroid hormone (TH) is the principle hormone that regulates our production of energy, our metabolism, our temperature, and our heart rate. It must be available in its optimum amount for us to have optimum health.

Thyroid hormones are the source of our vitality and youth.

Thyroid hormone is secreted by the thyroid gland that is positioned in the base of the neck. It regulates our metabolism by controlling the production of energy in our cells. The fuel from food and stored fat combines with oxygen in our cells to produce the chemical energy that powers all the functions of our body from movement to thought. The thyroid hormone, thyroxin, is the regulator of this process and the controller of our body heat and rate of cellular activity.

In normal, healthy people the thyroid hormone builds up with age ant then, almost always, begins to decline – for most people – in late middle age. When it begins to decline with age or for some other reason, our metabolism is slowed down.

The slowing of our metabolism causes the following problems:

Fatigue and loss of energy
Weakness
Susceptible to colds and viruses
Heavier, and more labored breathing
Muscle cramps
Persistent low back pain
Bruising easily
Mental sluggishness, poor memory
Headaches
Emotional instability
Cold hands and feet
Dry, course, or leathery, or pale skin
Course hair or loss of hair

Brittle nails
Stiff joints
Reduced interest in sex
Clogged arteries
Poor circulation

If the thyroid is not secreting enough hormones, there will not be enough energy or stamina. This condition is called myxedema (hypothyroidism).

The imbalance of thyroid hormones may also be responsible for disorders such as arteriosclerosis, high blood pressure, and senility among people who are not very old.

If there is an excess secretion of thyroid hormones, as in Basedow's disease (also known as Graves' disease), there will be too much energy. The body will be quickly worn out as the "throttle" is wide open for too long.

Eating too much kelp, for example, may trigger Basedow's disease because kelp contains a large amount of substances that make up thyroid hormones.

During the heavy bombing of London during World War II, an unusually high number of people in London were affected by Basedow's disease. At the onset of the Gulf War, President Bush was affected by Basedow's disease. The illness also affected Mrs. Bush, and even their dog.

Basedow's disease is known as "war disease" because the extreme tension in the face of an enemy's attack may trigger the illness. This is another illustration of how stresses in our life can erode the balance of hormones.

Among young women, 1 in 20 to 30 is found to have an abnormality with the thyroid hormone.

Basedow's disease, Harshimoto's disease (hypothyroidism), and thyroid cancer are found more often among young women than men. Women are 5 times more likely to have abnormalities in their thyroid gland. This is because the thyroid gland and female hormones are closely related.

As an interesting side note, it is reported that among some tribes of American Indians, a bride's neck is measured to indicate how happy she is. Medically speaking, it makes sense to measure the neck for feelings of happiness or euphoria, for the neck may slightly increase in width as the thyroid responds to human feelings, swelling slightly as it produces hormones. Most of the supermodels that our young girls admire tend to be tall and thin, and have long, slender necks.

However, if you check the impressionist paintings of beautiful women or the Ukiyoe paintings of Japanese women, you will find women with fuller necks. It seems likely that women with high intelligence, warmth, and friendliness tend to have fuller necks because their thyroid glands are working actively.

Some people born with thyroid glands that do not function properly have been classified as mentally disabled. When given hormone supplements, many have shown remarkable progress. Their eyes become brighter, hair begins to grow, and they look more alert. This kind of treatment has gone beyond the experimental stage and is practiced clinically.

Studies have shown that more than 40% of the U.S. population is deficient in TH and therefore they suffer from some of the symptoms listed above.

They are also more susceptible to adult onset diabetes, Alzheimer's, memory problems, loss of concentration, and other forms of dementia. And many suffer various forms of depression and almost always are over weight. And, their cholesterol and triglycerides are abnormally high.

1) Benefits of Thyroid Hormone HRT

But, when TH is restored to youthful levels, these symptoms almost always cease – and many times the related diseases abate.

The Neurology Journal and *The Southern Medical Journal* have both reported cases in which TH supplements even reversed certain types of cancer. While there is not yet enough evidence to prove these benefits, investigations in this area are continuing.

2) Adverse Side Effects of Thyroid Hormone HRT

Too much TH will cause problems, specifically osteoporosis, and especially so in women. However, a carefully tailored dose program can insure that proper doses are not exceeded.

3) Thyroid Hormone Levels

Thyroid hormone levels are the same for both men and women. The levels build up to about age 55 and then sharply begin to decrease as we get older.

Age	Percent of Peak
0	0
5	39
10	66
15	71
30	96
55	100
70	41
75	29
90	8
120	0

4) Thyroid Hormone Precursors:

The precursors for thyroid hormone are as follows:

Supplement	Dose
L – Tyrosine	500 mg 2x/day
Vitamin B complex	100 mg 3x/day
Vitamin B2	50 mg 2x/day
Iodine	120 mcg per day
Beta – Carotene	5,000 IU 3x/day
Vitamin C	500 mg 3x/day
Vitamin E	400 IU 1x/day
Zinc	50 mg 1x/day

L-Tyrosine is an amino acid that provides building blocks, the B complex vitamins provides nutritional support, B2 is riboflavin, a critical building block, and vitamins C and E and beta-carotene provide antioxidant properties.

All of these, when taken with zinc, which is required for cell nuclei formation, and the fatty acids which are normally provided by diet, for cell membrane formation, provide the body with the building blocks needed for physical and mental development, protection, and healing.

Their abundance stimulates the thyroid to secrete sufficient TH to use these materials to perform its function of regulating metabolism, controlling temperature, and maintaining our immune system.

Chapter 10
Insulin

We would be remiss not to address the very important hormone, Insulin even though we do not include it in our discussion. It is the hormone that facilitates the transport of blood sugar, glucose, into our cells for fuel. It is normally released when we eat. Some glucose gets stored in the liver and muscles as glycogen, a complex carbohydrate that the body can call upon to meet energy needs. If insulin is not doing its job properly, then the excess glucose is more easily stored as fat and the break down of fat for energy is also impaired.

Insulin frequently becomes a hormonal problem as we get older; the body uses it less efficiently and the resulting condition, called insulin resistance, is associated with increased obesity, high blood pressure, and cardiovascular risk. Careful diet and exercise can minimize the problem, but insulin HRT is frequently required.

Precise monitoring devices and techniques have been developed to measure glucose levels in the blood of diabetics and borderline diabetics. General speaking, glucose levels of less than 99 micrograms per deciliter of blood are considered normal, over 130 diabetic, and in between, borderline diabetic.

One can become diabetic as insulin resistance builds with age – as mentioned above – or when the Laggerhorn glands of the pancreas fail to produce sufficient insulin. Defective genes that cause, or allow, the immune system to attack and destroy the Laggerhorn, usually cause the later. This form of diabetics is termed Type I, or "juvenile on-set diabetics." The diabetics that starts as we age, is termed Type II, or "adult on-set diabetics".

Either form of diabetics requires insulin HRT for survival. Insulin HRT is the second largest (after estrogen) HRT program in use today. Genetically altered bacteria manufacture 97% of the insulin used in the U.S.A. These bacteria have had human gene that instructs for the manufacture of human insulin, spliced into their chromosomes.

We do not address the insulin and diabetics issues because detailed programs have been established and diabetic treatments are generally well established.

Chapter 11
Stress Hormones

There are many other hormones that control various aspects of our daily functions. We would be remiss in not mentioning them even though we do not include them in our detailed discussions.

1) Adrenaline

Adrenaline is made by noradrenalin, and the two hormones work together like twins. Adrenaline is the hormone released instantaneously when we experience fear or danger; it is a conditional reflex.

Adrenaline prepares our body and mind for emergency actions. However, the release of adrenaline is like an explosion, and it does not last.

Adrenaline can enable us to accomplish incredible things, but it cannot maintain this ability, and its effects disappear within a few minutes.

Suppose you're walking across the street when suddenly a run-away truck comes roaring your way. You leap across the distance separating you from the sidewalk, and it misses you by inches. You notice that you are trembling, that your heart is pounding, that your physical reaction is entirely out of proportion to the physical effort you just made. In fact, you are dealing with an adrenaline surge, which he body was able to send forth in time it took you to save your life.

Adrenaline is simply one of the most spectacular of the body's key hormones. It provides the sudden surge of energy needed for the severe cases of stress.

This hormone evolved in our pre-human ancestors so they would have the added energy for "fight or flight." Our biggest problem with it now is that it is frequently secreted we are under our new world stresses: stresses that last hours rather than the almost instance stresses for which they were originally designed in our ancestors.

2) Other Stress Hormones

Our body's reaction to adrenaline, and other so-called "stress hormones", and indeed to a great variety of hormones secreted by the Pituitary, hypothalamic glands, and many other secretions from localized Pituitary Hormones, and from Hypothalamic Hormones glands, are major contributors to a person's health profile.

While most HRT programs do not generally administer these hormones, it is vital that their levels be periodically monitored to properly assess the health profile of aging individuals.

Stress is one of the major causes of the rate of increased aging. See **Aging is a Treatable Disease** and my website **UnknownTruths.com**.

Conclusions

Our hormones are essential for body functions. However their needed levels decrease with age. Tests have shown that we can take supplements and injections (HRT) to return the decreasing levels to more youthful levels. But there can be adverse side effects.

It is safer to use precursor supplements to provide the ingredients (HPT) for the body to increase production of the needed hormone levels.

All of these findings and procedures are too new for the Government to give total approval. It will take time and more results to define the best way to personally tailor protocols suitable for each individual who is in need of hormone replacement or enhancement of hormone production in the body.

One such program is currently undergoing the needed tests and it is believed by the author that it will prove effective. When the results are in they will be published by the author in a new book: **Aging is Preventable**.

About the Author

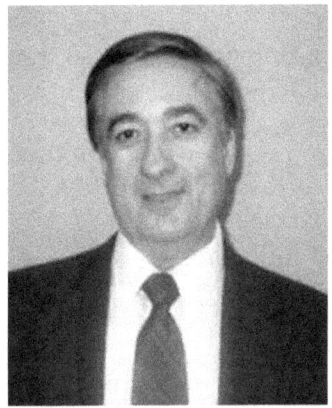

Hi! Thanks so much for your interest in my books!

My principal interests are true stories of the unusual or of the previously Unknown or unexplained. I have occasionally also written some fiction.

I was born in Memphis Tennessee and grew up in a small town near Tupelo Mississippi.

After graduating from Mississippi State University as an aerospace engineer I moved to Orlando Florida and worked for Lockheed Martin for 24 years. I advanced from an aerospace engineer to a Vice President of the Company and President of the Tactical Weapons Systems Division.

I then formed Parks-Jaggers Aerospace Company and sold it 4 years later.

I continued my education throughout my career with a MBA degree from Rollins College and with Post Graduate Studies in Astrophysics at UCLA; Laser Physics at the University of Michigan; Computer Science at the University of Florida; and Finance and Accounting at the Wharton School, University of Pennsylvania.

After selling my aerospace company I formed Quest Studios, Quest Entertainment and Rosebud Entertainment to make films at

Universal Studios. I produced 10 films, directed 7 films and wrote 5 films produced at Universal Studios.

I then formed UnknownTruths Publishing Company to publish true stories of the unusual or of the previously Unknown or unexplained. These include books about past events so unbelievable that most people have relegated them to "myths".

I have published 22 books as previously listed and have an additional 12 in development including the following:

Aging is Preventable describes how our new knowledge of the human aging process and supplementation protocols can essentially stop aging.

Female Sex, Orgasm and Love describes the science of the female sex process and the hormones and physical events resulting in true love.

End of Honor, Death of the Mafia is a true story about how the Mafia lost its honor when its members talked during the Rudy Giuliani trials.

Federal Rat describes the true story of the life and capers of a career criminal and how he manipulated the Federal Justice System to keep getting out of prison and returning to his life of crime.

Crystal Healing describes the science of (potentially) healing crystals.

Shakma, Filming a Crazed Baboon describes the frustrating experience of making the film Shakma at Universal Studios with a crazed baboon.

Eden Evolution addresses the question: how did mankind really get started; was there a Garden of Eden?

Cain's Wife addresses the dichotomy between the Biblical story of how mankind started with Adam and Eve in the Garden of Eden and scientific evidence of evolution.

Sex in the Ancient Churches describes how the ancients recognized that sex and the sun produced life and how they used it in their rituals and places of worship.

How to Make a Zombie describes the science of how to make a true zombie and describes actual instances.

Dam I Didn't Know That describes interesting tidbits that most people do not know but are important enough to know.

Alien Arrival, the First Visit is a novel about alien encounters through the ages, and today.

About
UnKnownTruths
Publishing Company

UnKnownTruths Publishing Company was formed to publish true stories of the unusual or of the previously Unknown or unexplained. These stories typically provide radically different views from those that have shaped the understandings of our natural world, our religions, our science, our history, and even the foundations of our civilizations.

The Company's stories also include stories of the very important anti-aging, life-extending medical breakthroughs; stem cell therapies; genetic therapies; cloning and other emerging findings that promise to change the very meaning of life.

The Company also publishes stories from the past that are so unbelievable that they are generally considered to be myths. The published stories provide the evidence for the truth.

The Company currently has an additional 12 books in development.

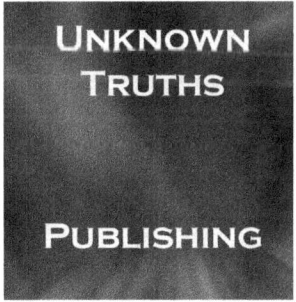